NursetoNurse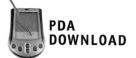

PALLIATIVE CARE

FOLLOW THESE INSTRUCTIONS TO DOWNLOAD YOUR PDA SOFTWARE

1) Use your Web browser to go to:
   http://www.mhnursetonurse.com

2) Register now

3) Fill in the required fields

4) Enter your unique registration code below

5) Download the software and sync into your handheld device

Code Listed Here

5948d587

Use this code to register and receive your PDA software. See above for complete directions.

If you have any problems accessing your download, please email: techsolutions@mhedu.com

ISBN 978-0-07-159086-0
MHID 0-07-159086-2
part of set
ISBN 978-0-07-149323-9
MHID 0-07-149323-9

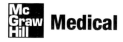

mcgraw-hillmedical.com

Nurse to Nurse
PALLIATIVE CARE

Nurse to Nurse: Palliative Care

1 2 3 4 5 6 7 8 9 0   DOC/DOC   12 11 10 9 8

Set ISBN 978-0-07-149323-9; MHID 0-07-149323-9
Book ISBN 978-0-07-159085-3; MHID 0-07-159085-4
PDA card ISBN 978-0-07-159086-0; MHID 0-07-159086-2

This book was set in Berkeley Book by International Typesetting and Composition.
The editors were Quincy McDonald and Karen Davis.
The production supervisor was Catherine H. Saggese.
Production management was provided by Preeti Longia Sinha, International Typesetting and Composition.
The book designer was Eve Siegel.
The cover designer was David Dell'Accio.
The index was prepared by Susan Hunter.
RR Donnelley was printer and binder.

This book is printed on acid-free paper.

Library of Congress Cataloging-in-Publication Data

Campbell, Margaret L., 1954-
    Nurse to nurse. Palliative care / Margaret L. Campbell.
        p. ; cm.
    Includes bibliographical references and index.
    ISBN-13: 978-0-07-149323-9 (pbk. : alk. paper)
    ISBN-10: 0-07-149323-9 (pbk. : alk. paper)
    1. Palliative treatment.   2. Terminal care.   3. Nursing.   I. Title.
    II. Title: Palliative care.
    [DNLM: 1. Nursing Staff, Hospital.   2. Palliative Care.   3. Nursing
    Care. 4.   Professional-Family Relations. WY 152 C189n 2009]
    RT87.T45C36 2009
    616'.029—dc22
                                                            2008025391

This book is respectfully dedicated to every nurse who brings knowledge, skill, and compassion to the care of terminally ill patients and their families

Contents

Contents

Preface

Since I entered nursing practice I have seen many changes in how dying patients are cared for in the hospital. I recall when DNR orders were rare and regardless of age, diagnosis, or prognosis we attempted to resuscitate anyone who was found without vital signs, even when we knew intuitively that it was unlikely to work. I also recall deferring all patient or family questions to the physician even when the answer was apparent to me and my colleagues; we had to make patients wait until the physician was available.

Once life supports were initiated, the patient remained on them until death regardless of level of consciousness or burden. The only end-of-life training I received in my basic nursing program was how to complete postmortem care.

Today, nurses practice in collaboration with physicians; resuscitation is rarely attempted when the poor prognosis is known; burdensome and nonbeneficial treatments are routinely withheld and withdrawn; ethics committees guide standards of practice; and there is a growing body of evidence to guide clinical care. Most schools and colleges of nursing provide content about the palliative care and care at the end of life, not just how to bag and tag the body. The National Institute of Nursing Research at the NIH holds the portfolio for end-of-life research.

This book is intended for the hospital nurse caring for patients who may be approaching the end of life. The practical tips and strategies and communication suggestions may enhance previous training and/or experience. Whether the patient is discharged for continued care in the community or dies in the hospital, the nurse is integral to providing comprehensive care. It is my hope that every hospital-based nurse will have basic knowledge and skills to care for any patient on any unit who needs aggressive symptom treatment or may be dying. Someday, when it's my turn to face the end of life I expect to find that every nurse who engages with me and my family will be skillful and compassionate.

Acknowledgments

This book would not have been possible without the support, encouragement, and constructive advice from editors and staff at McGraw-Hill, especially Quincy McDonald, Acquisition Editor. Likewise, my friends, family, and spouse, Michael Czechowski, give me space when I need it to write, and rewrite, and rewrite. I thank you all.

List of Acronyms

ADLs	activities of daily living
ALS	amyotrophic lateral sclerosis
AND	Allow Natural Death
ATS	American Thoracic Society
CHF	congestive heart failure
CMS	Centers for Medicare and Medicaid services
COPD	chronic obstructive pulmonary disease
CPR	cardiopulmonary resuscitation
DCD	Donation after Cardiac Death
DNR	Do Not Resuscitate
ED	emergency department
FAST	Functional Assessment Staging Tool
FEV1	Forced Expiratory Volume at 1 second
GOLD	Global Initiative for COPD
HF	heart failure
ICD	Implantable cardioverter defibrillator
ICU	intensive care unit
IR	immediate release
JCAHO	Joint Commission on Accreditation of Healthcare Organizations
MS	multiple sclerosis
NCP	National Consensus Project
NICU	Neurologic Intensive Care Unit
NSAID	nonsteroidal anti-inflammatory drug
OPO	Organ Procurement Organization
OR	operating room
PCU	Palliative Care Unit
PEG	percutaneous endoscopic gastrostomy
PPS	Palliative Performance Scale
SR	sustained release
VAS	Visual analog scale

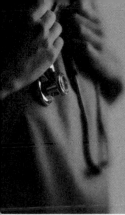

Chapter 1

NURSE'S ROLE IN PROVIDING CARE TO DYING PATIENTS

Stella Kowalski, RN, BSN, is a new graduate who has just completed hospital orientation. She has begun a rotation to the night shift and is in charge of an 18-bed medical-surgical unit with one other RN and two nurses' aides. During change of shift report she learns about Mr. Evans. He is an 80-year-old man admitted that evening from the nursing home with UTI and bacteremia complicating his advanced stage Alzheimer disease. His wife is at his bedside and plans to spend the night.

Stella observes an order in Mr. Evans's chart for "DNR—comfort measures only." Stella has no experience with terminal illness and was out sick the day her class made hospice visits when she was a junior. In Mr. Evans's chart, Stella notes a consult request for palliative care for advice about symptom management and a case manager consult to coordinate a hospice referral at discharge. Neither the palliative care consultant nor the case manager has seen the patient yet.

? Frequently Asked Questions

- What does DNR mean for my patient?
- What can I say to the family?
- Are there standards for care of dying patients?
- What is palliative care?

• What can I expect from a palliative care team consult?
• What is hospice care?

WHAT DOES DNR MEAN FOR MY PATIENT?

DNR is an acronym that stands for Do Not Resuscitate. DNR means do not attempt to use cardiopulmonary resuscitation (CPR) at the time of patient's death. Sometimes a DNR order carries other meanings. For example, prior to patient death, DNR might mean "Do not transfer to ICU" or "Do not intubate" or "Do not use aggressive life-saving measures." In some cases DNR means "comfort measures only." Some hospitals have shifted from DNR to AND which stands for Allow Natural Death.

It is critical that the nurse understand the treatment *goals* associated with the individual patient's DNR or AND order. Some patients with DNR orders will get full, aggressive treatment of potentially reversible illnesses or complications but no CPR if they die in spite of treatment. For other patients with DNR orders, the goal is to focus on comfort. The nursing care prior to death of a patient with DNR orders will be dependent on the treatment goals. Collaboration with the patient's physician is an essential component for clarification of the patient's treatment goals with DNR. Clear documentation of the treatment goals is essential so that all clinical staff understand the treatment plan.

Mr. Evans's order reads "DNR-comfort measures only." This means that the only treatments Mr. Evans will receive are those that promote comfort. He will not be resuscitated if he dies during the night and, prior to death as his vital signs and breathing change, he will not receive any heroic measures such as intubation or vasopressors. Mr. Evans will receive treatments to minimize or eliminate any distress.

For more information about the nurse's role and DNR decisions see the American Nurses Association (ANA) position statement in Appendix A.

 Clinical Alert
DNR (Do Not Resuscitate) or AND (Allow Natural Death) orders are incomplete without clarification of the treatment goals (e.g., comfort measures only).

WHAT CAN I SAY TO THE FAMILY?

Communication with the patient and family is a standard of professional nursing practice. According to the American Nurses Association *Scope and Standards of Practice* (2004),[1] the registered nurse:

- Communicates with patient, family, and health-care providers regarding patient care and the nurse's role in the provision of that care.

  For example, clarification of Mr. Evans's treatment goals with the nurse from the afternoon shift and with the patient's wife typifies this standard.

- Collaborates in creating a documented plan, focused on outcomes and decisions related to care and delivery of services, which indicates communication with patients, families, and others.

The earliest study of the needs of spouses of patients dying in the hospital revealed that communication needs were the most important.[2] Spouses reported the need for:

- Assurance of the comfort of the patient
- Information about the patient's condition
- Information about the impending death

The nurse will be most successful communicating with families of dying patients if she or he:

- Reinforces interdisciplinary communication
- Ensures that physicians are aware of communication gaps
- Listens as much as speaks
- Acknowledges emotions
- Makes assurances about patient comfort

 Clinical Alert
Family stress increases when frequent communication from nurses and physicians is lacking.

Chapter 4 provides more detail about communication with patients and their families.

ARE THERE STANDARDS FOR CARE OF DYING PATIENTS?

Standards reflect the values and priorities of the professions who care for the dying. A national collaboration of experts in dying care produced the National Consensus Project (NCP) for Quality Palliative Care. The purpose of the NCP for Quality Palliative Care is to promote the implementation of *Clinical Practice Guidelines for Quality Palliative Care* that ensure care of consistent and high quality, and that guide the development and structure of new and existing palliative care services.[3]

The guidelines describe core precepts and structures of clinical palliative care programs divided into eight dedicated sections:

1. Structure and Processes of Care
2. Physical Aspects of Care

3. Psychological and Psychiatric Aspects of Care
4. Social Aspects of Care
5. Spiritual, Religious, and Existential Aspects of Care
6. Cultural Aspects of Care
7. Care of the Imminently Dying Patient
8. Ethical and Legal Aspects of Care

How to Say It

Assurance of patient comfort
"The medication I just gave your husband will start to work in about 20 minutes. I'll be back to check that he gets relief."
"I don't see any signs of pain or shortness of breath. His face muscles are relaxed, his breathing pattern is normal, and he's sleeping. That tells me he's comfortable."

Information about the patient's condition
"His blood pressure is lower today than yesterday. That means he's getting closer to dying."
"His hands and feet are cooler because his blood pressure dropped. This doesn't cause any distress for him."

Information about the impending death
"Mrs. Evans, your husband has made some changes that tell me he is close to dying. You should stay nearby or in his room if you want to be with him when he dies."

Reinforce interdisciplinary communication
"What has the physician told you today? I'll see if I can explain it."

Acknowledge emotions
"I can see that I've made you cry."
"You seem more upset today than yesterday."
"You look like you might be angry. Has something upset you?"

The interested nurse may download the full text document or the executive summary of the NCP Guidelines at www. nationalconsensusproject.org. (See Appendix B for an excerpt from the Executive Summary of the NCP Guidelines.) The National Quality Forum built on the NCP Guidelines by identifying preferred practices for palliative and hospice care quality. These guidelines are available for purchase at http:// www.qualityforum.org/publications/reports/palliative.asp. Six preferred practices for care of the imminently dying patient are described in a publication by Lynch and Dahlin.[4]

In addition to the aforementioned standards, some nursing organizations have published position papers relevant to care of the dying. The following position statements from the **American Nurses Association** are included in the appendices:

- Nursing Care and Do-Not-Resuscitate Orders (Appendix A)
- Pain Management and Care of Distressing Symptoms in Dying Patients (Appendix C)

The following position statements from the **Hospice and Palliative Nurses Association** are included in the appendices and are accessible at www.hpna.org:

- Value of Professional Nurse in End-of-Life Care (Appendix D)
- Providing Opioids at End of Life (Appendix E)
- Artificial Nutrition and Hydration in End-of-Life Care (Appendix F)
- Complementary Therapies (Appendix G)
- Spiritual Care (Appendix H)

The **Oncology Nursing Society** position statement, "Oncology Nursing Society and Association of Oncology Social Work Joint Position on End-of-Life Care," is accessible at www.ons.org/publications/positions.

WHAT IS PALLIATIVE CARE?

Several definitions of palliative care exist but have similar concepts. **The World Health Organization (WHO)** states: "Palliative care improves the quality of life of patients and families

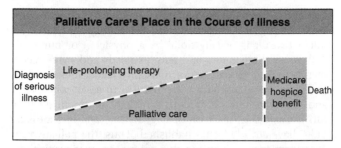

Figure 1-1 Conceptualization of palliative care integration across illness course. (Reproduced with permission from National Consensus Project for Quality Palliative Care, Pittsburg, PA, www.nationalconsensusproject.org.)

who face life-threatening illness, by providing pain and symptom relief, spiritual and psychosocial support from diagnosis to the end of life and bereavement" (www.who.int/ cancer/palliative/en). Palliative care is defined by the **National Consensus Project for Quality Palliative Care** thus:

> The goal of palliative care is to prevent and relieve suffering and to support the best possible quality of life for patients and their families, regardless of the stage of the disease or the need for other therapies. Palliative care is both a philosophy of care and an organized, highly structured system for delivering care. Palliative care expands traditional disease-model medical treatments to include the goals of enhancing quality of life for patients and family, optimizing function, helping with decision making and providing opportunities for personal growth. As such, it can be delivered concurrently with life-prolonging care or as the main focus of care (Figure 1-1).

WHAT CAN I EXPECT FROM A PALLIATIVE CARE TEAM CONSULT?

Palliative care teams in hospitals are typically interdisciplinary and usually include a physician and/or an advanced practice nurse along with support from one or more social workers and chaplains. Additionally, the team may use the services of

colleagues from dietary and rehabilitation, such as occupational or physical therapists, and respiratory therapists. The
initial consult is usually done by a physician or nurse who
will assess the patient's and family's needs and make recommendations to the patient's primary physician. Sometimes, the
palliative care consultant is brought in to assist with patient
and family communication to establish treatment goals. In
Mr. Evans's case, the treatment goals for "comfort measures
only" have already been established. Thus, the palliative care
consultant may be advising about symptom management and
hospice discharge eligibility. Additionally, the consultant may
advise how to support the patient's wife as she prepares for
the loss of her husband.

Usually, the patient's primary physician, if there is one, continues to see the patient and write orders. The palliative care
consultant may also see the patient and write advisory notes or
write orders depending on the collaborative relationship with
the primary physician. In some hospitals the patient's care might
be transferred to the palliative care team, and the admitting
physician "signs off." Palliative care consultants also provide
education to the hospital staff, especially novices who are inexperienced with care of dying patients.

In some cases there are disagreements among the patient's
family or with the physician or among members of the healthcare team about treatment goals when the patient is dying. A
palliative care consultant can be a useful mediator to reconcile
disagreements among parties and achieve unanimity about the
patient's care.

WHAT IS HOSPICE CARE?

Hospice care shares the same philosophy as palliative care.
However, "all hospice care is palliative care but not all palliative care
is hospice care."[5] Palliative care should be offered to any patient in
need of such services but hospice care is regulated and a patient
must have an expected survival of less than six months to
receive hospice care under the Medicare benefit (see Appendix I).

As with palliative care, hospice care is delivered using an interdisciplinary team model usually in the patient's home or a facility such as a nursing home. In some communities, free-standing hospice facilities provide another optional setting. Some hospitals have collaborative agreements to provide hospital care to the hospice patient when aggressive symptom management is needed, or when the patient is actively dying, or when respite is needed by the family. The nurse can learn more about hospice care from the **National Hospice and Palliative Care Organization** at www.nhpco.org.

CLOSING VIGNETTE

Stella makes her rounds and when she introduces herself to Mrs. Evans, she says, "I'm Ms. Kowalski and I will be taking care of your husband tonight. I understand that our goal is to keep him comfortable. I also want to be of help to you, tonight. I'm still a new nurse, but I'll do my best, especially if you tell me how I can help you. The palliative care specialists will see your husband in the morning."

Throughout the night, Stella checks on Mr. and Mrs. Evans each time she passes the room. She is uncertain about how frequently she should turn him and about the care of his decubitus ulcers. She plans to ask her colleagues in the morning during report.

Mr. Evans needs his prescribed pain medication only once and Mrs. Evans dozes in the chair by the bed. Stella has gotten her a blanket from the linen cart and soup and crackers from the unit pantry.

CLOSING PEARL

Even an inexperienced nurse has core assessment skills and core family coping skills to ensure that a dying patient and his family are well cared for.

REFERENCES

1. American Nurses Association. *Scope and Standards of Practice*. Washington, DC: American Nurses Association; 2004.
2. Hampe SO. Needs of the grieving spouse in a hospital setting. *Nursing Research*. 1975;24:113–120.
3. National Consensus Project for Quality Palliative Care. *Clinical Practice Guidelines for Quality Palliative Care*. Brooklyn, NY: 2004.
4. Lynch M, Dahlin CM. The National Consensus Project and National Quality Forum preferred practices in care of the imminently dying patient. *Journal of Hospice and Palliative Nursing*. 2007;9(6):316–322.
5. Fischberg D, Morris J, Avellanet C. Palliative care. In: Panke JT, Coyne P, eds. *Conversations in Palliative Care*. 2nd ed. Pittsburgh, PA: Hospice and Palliative Nurses Association; 2006:1–8.

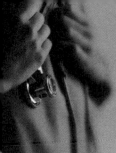

Chapter 2
PATIENT PROGNOSIS

William Jackson, RN, BSN, is an experienced medical-surgical staff nurse and he is the case manager for a 16-bed medical unit. His unit is not specialized and largely admits patients with medical illnesses although surgical overflow patients are also admitted. William is making rounds with the unit charge nurse to identify patients who may have special needs at discharge (Table 2-1).

? Frequently Asked Questions

- How is terminal illness defined?
- How do I know when a patient is terminally ill?
- Are the terminal illness trajectories the same for all diagnoses?
- How do I know when a patient is close to death?
- Does a patient have to be in the hospital when he or she dies?

HOW IS TERMINAL ILLNESS DEFINED?

Terminal illness is a difficult term to define. It is generally understood to mean that a person has an incurable illness that is expected to progress to death. Medicare has defined a terminal illness, for purposes of hospice enrollment, as a predicted lifespan of less than 6 months. Patients might define the terminal stage as "when I have to be in bed and can no longer care for myself."

Some incurable illnesses have a longer natural life-span than others and patient choices about the use of life-sustaining

Table 2-1 Unit Census with Patient Age, Name, and Admitting Diagnosis

Age	Name	Diagnosis	Age	Name	Diagnosis
38	Tyrone	Pneumonia	72	Miles	CHF exacerbation
48	George	DKA	69	Sharon	Ischemic stroke
24	Tina	Multiple fractures	88	Willie Mae	UTI, dehydration
43	Timothy	Pancreatic cancer	78	Harold	COPD exacerbation
86	Clarence	Anemia, lower GI bleed, advanced dementia	50	Jack	Asthma
62	Frank	Lung cancer	48	Jeanne	Acute renal failure
70	Louise	CHF exacerbation	68	Victor	Seizures
92	Gertrude	Pneumonia	36	John	Infected decubiti, paraplegia

treatments or technologies or organ transplantation will change the illness trajectory. For example, patients who are anuric with end-stage renal disease can live for years with dialysis, but for less than 2 weeks if they refuse dialysis. Thus, the age or diagnosis of the patient taken alone does not provide enough information to identify who is terminally ill.

As he returns to the unit census, William may want to look more closely at the highlighted patients for evidence of an underlying terminal illness. The age and admitting diagnosis may give a clue but do not give enough information to conclude that any of these patients have reached the terminal stage of their illnesses (Table 2-2).

Table 2-2 Unit Census with Patients at Risk for Terminal Illness Highlighted

Age	Name	Diagnosis	Age	Name	Diagnosis
38	Tyrone	Pneumonia	72	Miles	CHF exacerbation
48	George	DKA	69	Sharon	Ischemic stroke
24	Tina	Multiple fractures	88	Willie Mae	UTI, dehydration
43	Timothy	Pancreatic cancer	78	Harold	COPD exacerbation
86	Clarence	Anemia, lower GI bleed, advanced dementia	50	Jack	Asthma
62	Frank	Lung cancer	48	Jeanne	Acute renal failure
70	Louise	CHF exacerbation	68	Victor	Seizures
92	Gertrude	Pneumonia	36	John	Infected decubiti, paraplegia

HOW DO I KNOW WHEN A PATIENT IS TERMINALLY ILL?

A nurse may begin an assessment for terminal illness by looking at the patient's admitting diagnosis and perhaps age, but a review of the medical record will provide a more complete patient description. The nurse should look for evidence of the following, usually found in the History and Physical Examination section of the medical record:

• Characterization of the illness stage

— Are any terms such as advanced, end stage, or terminal used?

- Patient treatment goals
  — Are treatment goals such as DNR identified?
  — Are patient preferences for use of life supports documented?
  — Is surgery, chemotherapy, or radiation planned?
  — Is the patient a candidate for organ transplantation?

William reviews the medical record of Timothy, the 43-year-old patient with pancreatic cancer. He notes that the patient had an exploratory laparotomy that revealed carcinomatosis (extensive metastatic lesions) that could not be resected surgically. He also reads the oncology consultant note that states that the cancer is terminal and no supportive treatment will change the outcome. The oncologist recommends referral to hospice.

When William reviews the record of Frank, the 62-year-old patient with lung cancer, he notes that the cancer is nonsmall cell type and localized to the right upper lobe (treatable). The patient is going to begin treatment with radiation.

We see there are two patients with cancer, but until the medical record for each is reviewed for stage and treatment options the nurse cannot conclude if either of these patients is terminal. Note that age is not a factor in this assessment.

 Clinical Alert
Age is not a reliable criterion for identifying patients who are approaching the end of life.

ARE THE TERMINAL ILLNESS TRAJECTORIES THE SAME FOR ALL DIAGNOSES?

A dying trajectory has two properties, duration and shape.[1] In a study of the patterns of dying of Medicare recipients

Death trajectories

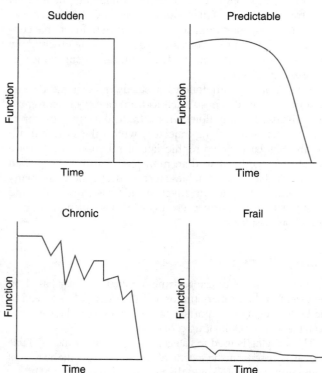

Figure 2-1 Prototypical terminal illness projectories.

investigators suggested four prototypical trajectories[2,3] (Figure 2-1).

A *sudden* death is unexpected and usually occurs outside the hospital, such as from accidents or trauma. Other causes of sudden death include myocardial infarction and hemorrhagic stroke; these occur from previously undiagnosed vascular disease. Because the patient dies suddenly the emphasis of care may be on the family if death is pronounced in the Emergency Department. (See Chapters 5 and 6 for family care considerations.)

Sometimes, the person who sustains a sudden death in the community has CPR attempted and is admitted to the hospital for a trial of ICU care. Often, out-of-hospital CPR is unsuccessful at producing long-term survival or return to functional consciousness [4,5] and decisions are frequently made to withdraw life-sustaining treatments.[6] This clinical circumstance is addressed in Chapter 6.

A *predictable* death follows a steady, predictable decline from the time of diagnosis such as from cancer or neuromuscular disease. The duration varies with the illness, for example, some cancers have a long trajectory while others cause death rapidly. Similarly, amyotrophic lateral sclerosis (ALS) has a shorter average lifespan than multiple sclerosis (MS). When the patient has a predictable cause of death there are many opportunities to plan in advance, address symptoms, and bring together supportive resources for the patient and family, such as hospice care.

Cancer Staging

Staging is a means of categorizing a patient's cancer based on the extent of the primary tumor and the extent of its spread in the body. Staging is important for determining if the cancer is treatable and for estimating prognosis.

TNM staging is used to categorize solid tumor cancers (Table 2-3). It is based on the extent of the tumor (T), the extent of lymph node spread (N), and the presence of metastasis (M).

Timothy's pancreatic cancer has been staged as T4N3M1. Frank's lung cancer is staged T1N0M0.

Overall stage grouping (Table 2-4) uses roman numerals to describe the progression of cancer.

Timothy's cancer is stage IV, but Frank's cancer is stage I.

For more detailed information about cancer staging go to the National Cancer Institute fact sheet at http://www.cancer.gov/cancertopics/factsheet/Detection/staging.

Death following *chronic* illness typifies the course for chronic obstructive pulmonary disease (COPD) and congestive heart

Table 2-3 TNM Staging of Solid Tumor Cancers

Tumor	
TX	Primary tumor cannot be evaluated
T0	No evidence of primary tumor
Tis	Tumor *in situ* (early cancer has not spread)
T1, T2, T3, T4	Size and/or extent of the primary tumor
Nodes	
NX	Regional lymph nodes cannot be evaluated
N0	No regional lymph node involvement
N1, N2, N3	Involvement of regional lymph nodes
Metastasis	
MX	Distant metastasis cannot be evaluated
M0	No distant metastasis
M1	Distant metastasis

Table 2-4 Overall Stage Grouping for Cancer

Stage 0	Cancer in situ
Stage I	Cancer is localized to one part of the body
Stage II–III	Cancer is locally advanced, the specific criteria for stages II and III differ by cancer type
Stage IV	Cancer has metastasized to other organs or throughout the body

failure (CHF). These diseases are not curable but there are supportive treatments and rescue treatments during acute exacerbations. For instance, patients with COPD from any cause may live with the condition for many years with supportive treatments including bronchodilators and oxygen. The later stage of chronic illness may produce exacerbations causing temporary hospitalization and even admission to the ICU with life supports such as mechanical ventilation. Often, the patients with CHF or COPD do not view themselves as terminal even though they have progressive, incurable diseases. Because these illnesses are less predictable it is more difficult to identify the terminal phase and refer the patient for palliative or hospice care. As we saw in Chapter 1, integration of palliative care along with supportive or prolongative treatment may improve the chronically ill patient's quality of life.

Heart Failure Staging

There are two commonly used approaches to the classification of heart failure (HF). The American Heart Association/American College of Cardiologists (AHA/ACC) classification emphasizes the progression of HF.[7] The New York Heart Association (NYHA) classification categorizes patients according to their functional capacity.[8] The two classification systems complement one another (Table 2-5).

Table 2-5   Classification of Heart Failure

AHA/ACC Stage		NYHA Functional Class	
Stage	Description	Class	Description
A	Patients at high risk of developing HF because of the presence of conditions strongly associated with the development of HF. Such patients have no identifiable structural or functional abnormalities of the pericardium, myocardium, or cardiac valves, and have never shown signs or symptoms of HF.		

(Continued)

Table 2-5 Classification of Heart Failure (*Continued*)

AHA/ACC Stage		NYHA Functional Class	
Stage	**Description**	**Class**	**Description**
B	Patients who have developed structural heart disease that is strongly associated with the development of HF but who have never shown signs or symptoms of HF.	I	No limitation of physical activity. Ordinary physical activity does not cause undue fatigue, palpitation, or dyspnea.
C	Patients who have current or prior symptoms of HF associated with underlying structural heart disease.	II	Slight limitation of physical activity. Comfortable at rest, but ordinary physical activity results in fatigue, palpitation, or dyspnea.
		III	Marked limitation of physical activity. Comfortable at rest, but less than ordinary activity causes fatigue, palpitation, or dyspnea.
D	Patients with advanced structural heart disease and marked symptoms of HF at rest despite maximal medical therapy and who require specialized interventions.	IV	Unable to carry out any physical activity without discomfort. Symptoms of cardiac insufficiency at rest. If any physical activity is undertaken, discomfort is increased.

From the AHA/ACC[7] and the NYHA in the Criteria Committee of the NYHA[8].

Louise has exertional dyspnea following a myocardial infarction. Her HF is an AHA/ACC stage C and NYHA stage II. However, Miles wears oxygen continuously and is unable to move from the bed to the bedside commode without becoming severely dyspneic. His HF is AHA/ACC stage D and NYHA stage IV.

Staging of COPD Severity

The single best predictor of COPD prognosis is the Forced Expiratory Volume at 1 second (FEV_1). It is expressed as a percentage of the total forced vital capacity. Both the American Thoracic Society (ATS)[9] and the Global Initiative for COPD (GOLD)[10] have proposed a 3-stage classification using the FEV_1 %; however, the criteria vary slightly (Table 2-6).

Harold uses oxygen as needed at home and is able to be independent with his activities of daily living. On a recent pulmonary function test his FEV_1 % was estimated at 45%, so although his disease is moderately severe he is not at the terminal stage.

A *frail* trajectory is characteristic of patients who have a poor functional status over a variable period of time without significant exacerbations. This trajectory represents patients with very advanced age, dementias, and those in a coma or vegetative state. The cause of death for patients in this trajectory

Table 2-6   Staging of COPD Severity

Severity	ATS[9]	GOLD[10]
	FEV_1 % predicted	
Stage 0: at risk	N/A	Normal
Stage 1: mild	≥50	>80
Stage 2: moderate	35–49	30–79
Stage 3: severe	<35	<30

N/A, not applicable.

is usually a complication from immobility, such as septic shock from a urinary tract infection or infected decubiti, or pneumonia.

Staging Alzheimer Disease

The Functional Assessment Staging Tool (FAST) is commonly used to categorize the course of Alzheimer disease.[11] Patients with advanced dementia are eligible for hospice referral if they are at the FAST level 7 and have one or more of dementia-associated comorbidities, such as aspiration, urinary tract infection, sepsis, multiple stage 3–4 ulcers, persistent fever, or weight loss >10% within six months (Figure 2-2).

1	Normal aging	No deficits whatsoever
2	Possible mild cognitive Impairment	Subjective functional deficit
3	Mild cognitive impairment	Objective function deficit Interferes with a person's most complex tasks
4	Mild dementia	IADLs become affected, such as bill paying, cooking, cleaning, traveling
5	Moderate dementia	Needs help selecting proper attire
6a	Moderately severe dementia	Needs help putting on clothes
6b	Moderately severe dementia	Needs help bathing
6c	Moderately severe dementia	Needs help toileting
6d	Moderately severe dementia	Urinary incontinence
6e	Moderately severe dementia	Fecal incontinence
7a	Severe dementia	Speaks 5–6 words during day
7b	Severe dementia	Speaks only 1 word clearly
7c	Severe dementia	Can no longer walk
7d	Severe dementia	Can no longer sit up
7e	Severe dementia	Can no longer smile
7f	Severe dementia	Can no longer hold up head

Figure 2-2 Functional assessment staging tool. From Reisberg (1988) with permission.

The FAST tool should be used to categorize a patient based on recent behavior. A patient who has an infection or is dehydrated may perform at a lower than normal level so it is important to ascertain the baseline FAST based on the patient's usual behavior before hospital admission.

Willie Mae was admitted with a UTI and dehydration. When the admission history and physical were obtained her daughter reported about Willie Mae's baseline functions. She could no longer manage her finances or cooking and cleaning. Willie Mae was confused at times but could still dress and bathe with minimal assistance and she sometimes needed help toileting but was only rarely incontinent of urine. Thus, Willie Mae is moderately severely demented at a FAST level 6d. Although, she does not meet hospice referral criterion this may be a good time to begin advance planning with the family.

Clarence, on the other hand, was admitted after his family noticed blood in his diaper after a bowel movement. At baseline, Clarence's family reported that Clarence was bed bound, nonverbal, and incontinent of urine and stool. On physical examination Clarence was found to have bilateral lower extremity contractures and a stage III right trochanter pressure ulcer. Clarence has severe dementia at FAST 7d and meets the hospice referral criterion.

Clinical Alert

Elderly and demented patients may decline rapidly from baseline functioning when sick. Assessment of baseline functional status must be done from usual behaviors displayed before the acute illness.

HOW DO I KNOW WHEN A PATIENT IS CLOSE TO DEATH?

We cannot say precisely how long a patient will live when he or she reaches the terminal stage. However, the following physical and neurologic changes occur as described for most patients.

Patients are close to death (days to weeks) when they

- lose the ability to perform activities of daily living without assistance
- lose an interest in food and drink
- sleep more than usual
- begin to display cognitive impairment (confusion, lethargy, delirium)

Death is imminent (<72 hours) when there is one or more signs of

- increased cognitive impairment, agitated delirium, or unconsciousness
- unstable vital signs
- no intake of food or drink
- decreased urine or stool
- pulmonary congestion, increased oropharyngeal secretions
- pallor, mottling, cyanosis
- peripheral edema, anasarca
- hypothermia
- cool extremities
- limited or no blinking
- altered breathing pattern (See Appendix J Breathing Patterns)
  — Cheyne-Stokes
  — Intrinsic medullary pattern (this occurs in patients with severe neurologic injuries)
  — Agonal (this pattern [not illustrated] looks like a fish out of water, patient's mouth is usually open and slow, occasional breaths are taken that produce little chest expansion, death usually follows in hours after this pattern is apparent)

Table 2-7 Palliative Performance Scale

PPS Level	Activity & Evidence of Ambulation	Disease	Self-Care	Intake	Conscious Level
100%	Full	Normal activity & work No evidence of disease	Full	Normal	Full
90%	Full	Normal activity & work Some evidence of disease	Full	Normal	Full
80%	Full	Normal activity *with* effort Some evidence of disease	Full	Normal or reduced	Full
70%	Reduced	Unable to do normal job/work Significant disease	Full	Normal or reduced	Full
60%	Reduced	Unable to do hobby/housework Significant disease	Occasional assistance necessary	Normal or reduced	Full or confusion
50%	Mainly sit/lie	Unable to do any work Extensive disease	Considerable assistance required	Normal or reduced	Full or confusion

40%	Mainly in bed	Unable to do most activity Extensive disease	Mainly assistance	Normal or reduced	Full or drowsy +/- confusion
30%	Totally bed bound	Unable to do any activity Extensive disease	Total care	Normal or reduced	Full or drowsy +/- confusion
20%	Totally bed bound	Unable to do any activity Extensive disease	Total care	Minimal to sips	Full or drowsy +/- confusion
10%	Totally bed bound	Unable to do any activity Extensive disease	Total care	Mouth care only	Drowsy or coma +/- confusion
0%	Death	—	—	—	—

Terminal illness severity has been quantified using the Palliative Performance Scale (PPS)[12] (Table 2-7). This scale grades a patient's general condition as 0% (dead) to 100% (normal) in increments of 10 percentage points. The scale incorporates five observer-rated parameters: ambulation, activity, self-care, intake, and level of consciousness. The scale has been validated with patients with cancer (all types), patients in an acute tertiary hospital setting, home care setting, and various diagnoses.[13–16]

Clarence is no longer taking oral intake and was bed bound with total care prehospital so his PPS score is 10%. Additionally, he is hypotensive, oliguric, hypothermic, and has audible retained upper airway secretions. There are no plans to work up the source of his GI bleeding since he is in the terminal stage of Alzheimer disease. Signs of imminent death (<72 hours) are evident.

DOES A PATIENT HAVE TO BE IN THE HOSPITAL WHEN HE OR SHE DIES?

A decision about the most optimal setting for a patient who is dying depends on several factors, including

* Imminence of death
* Complexity of care needs
* Availability of caregivers
  — Family
  — Professional
* Available settings
  — Hospital
  — Nursing home
  — Home
  — Hospice facility
* Access to palliative care resources, including hospice
* Patient or family preferences

A team approach to identifying the best setting is ideal. The patient's physician and nurse will have the expertise in identifying the dying trajectory and imminence of death along with interventions to meet the patient's care needs. The family will know their own abilities and access to other family resources. A hospital case manager, social worker, or discharge planner is the optimal colleague to advise about settings and community resources. Generally, except in the VA system, insurers will not reimburse hospitals for terminal care, thus, out-of-hospital settings need to be identified. When death is imminent, however, it is not compassionate to find a discharge option, unless the patient or family has strong desires for discharge. In some hospitals, there are beds designated for hospice care and the patient is discharged on paper and readmitted to hospice.

More information about finding hospice providers can be found at the National Hospice and Palliative Care Organization website (www.nhpco.org).

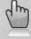

Clinical Alert

Resource utilization induced discharge is not appropriate when death is imminent unless the patient or family wants discharge.

CLOSING VIGNETTE

At the conclusion of his case-management rounds, William has identified three patients who are terminally ill although at different phases of dying. He has contacted the primary physicians for these patients and provided assistance in disposition to the optimal care setting. Death is expected in less than 3 days for Clarence, the 86-year-old patient with advanced dementia and lower GI bleeding, so he will stay in the hospital with palliative care treatment goals (Table 2–8).

Table 2-8 Unit Census, Patients with Terminal Disease

Age	Diagnosis	Name	Terminal?	Disposition
43	*Pancreatic cancer, carcinomatosis, stage IV, no planned radiation or chemotherapy*	*Timothy*	*Yes*	*Home hospice*
86	*Anemia, lower GI bleed, complicating advanced Alzheimer disease, no planned prolongative interventions*	*Clarence*	*Yes, imminent*	*Remain in hospital*
72	*CHF, NY Heart Association IV, ejection fraction 15%*	*Miles*	*Yes*	*Home hospice*

CLOSING PEARL

With knowledge about prognostication the nurse can be instrumental in assisting with disposition planning for terminally ill patients.

REFERENCES

1. Field MJ, Cassel CK, eds. *Approaching death: Improving care at the end of life.* Washington, D.C.: National Academy Press; 1997.
2. Lunney JR, Lynn J, Foley DJ, Lipson S, Guralnik JM. Patterns of functional decline at the end of life. *JAMA.* May 14 2003; 289(18):2387–2392.
3. Lunney JR, Lynn J, Hogan C. Profiles of older medicare decedents. *J Am Geriatr Soc.* Jun 2002;50(6):1108–1112.
4. Benkendorf R, Swor RA, Jackson R, Rivera-Rivera EJ, Demrick A. Outcomes of cardiac arrest in the nursing home: destiny or

futility? [see comment]. *Prehosp Emerg Care*. Apr–Jun 1997;1(2):68–72.

5. Dunne RB, Compton S, Zalenski RJ, Swor R, Welch R, Bock BF. Outcomes from out-of-hospital cardiac arrest in Detroit. *Resuscitation*. Jan 2007;72(1):59–65.

6. Booth CM, Boone RH, Tomlinson G, Detsky AS. Is this patient dead, vegetative, or severely neurologically impaired? Assessing outcome for comatose survivors of cardiac arrest. *JAMA*. Feb 18 2004;291(7):870–879.

7. Hunt SA, Baker DW, Chin MH, et al. ACC/AHA Guidelines for the Evaluation and Management of Chronic Heart Failure in the Adult: Executive Summary A Report of the American College of Cardiology/American Heart Association Task Force on Practice Guidelines (Committee to Revise the 1995 Guidelines for the Evaluation and Management of Heart Failure): Developed in Collaboration With the International Society for Heart and Lung Transplantation; Endorsed by the Heart Failure Society of America. *Circulation*. Dec 11 2001; 104(24):2996–3007.

8. The Criteria Committee of the New York Heart Association. Nomenclature and criteria for diagnosis of diseases of the heart and great vessels. 9th ed. Boston: Little, Brown & Co.; 1994:253–256.

9. American Thoracic Society. Standards for the diagnosis and care of patients with chronic obstructive pulmonary disease. *Am J Respir Crit Care Med*. 1995;152:S77–S121.

10. GOLD Expert Panel. Global Initiative for Chronic Obstructive Lung Disease. www.goldcopd.org.

11. Reisberg B. Functional assessment staging (FAST). *Psychopharmacol Bul*. 1988;24:653–659.

12. Anderson F, Downing GM, Hill J, Casorso L, Lerch N. Palliative performance scale (PPS): a new tool. *J Palliat Care*. Spring 1996;12(1):5–11.

13. Harrold J, Rickerson E, Carroll JT, et al. Is the palliative performance scale a useful predictor of mortality in a heterogeneous hospice population? *J Palliat Med*. Jun 2005; 8(3):503–509.

14. Head B, Ritchie CS, Smoot TM. Prognostication in hospice care: can the palliative performance scale help? *J Palliat Med.* Jun 2005;8(3):492–502.

15. Lau F, Downing GM, Lesperance M, Shaw J, Kuziemsky C. Use of Palliative Performance Scale in end-of-life prognostication. *J Palliat Med.* Oct 2006;9(5):1066–1075.

16. Olajide O, Hanson L, Usher BM, Qaqish BF, Schwartz R, Bernard S. Validation of the palliative performance scale in the acute tertiary care hospital setting. *J Palliat Med.* Feb 2007;10(1):111–117.

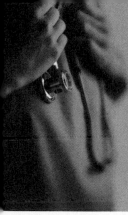

Chapter 3

PATIENT AND FAMILY NEEDS: EMPHASIS ON COMMUNICATION

Elsa Mitchell was admitted to the hospital directly from her doctor's office. She reported a 3-week history of worsening right upper quadrant pain that radiated to her back, nausea, jaundice, fatigue, and an unintentional 20-lb. weight loss. Her pancreatic and liver enzymes and bilirubin were significantly elevated and she was anemic and hypoalbuminemic. A CT scan of her abdomen was suggestive of widely metastatic pancreatic cancer. The consulting surgeon reported that the lesion was too extensive for surgical intervention. The oncologist recommended a palliative care consultation since the cancer was too advanced for treatment and Mrs. Mitchell was likely to die within 6 weeks. The primary physician broke this news to Mrs. Mitchell and her husband.

❓ Frequently Asked Questions

- What are the most common needs of the terminally ill patient?

- How should the nurse address patient needs for social connectedness, psychological distress, spirituality and patient-nurse relationship?

- What are the most common needs of the terminally ill patient's family?

- What is the nurse's role in communicating with patient or family about the patient's terminal illness?

- What are the communication needs of the dying patient's family?
- How should bad news be broken?
- How should treatment goals and DNR be discussed?
- How do these discussions occur when the patient has a dysfunctional family?
- What needs to happen if there is no mutual agreement about treatment goals?
- What can I tell patients and their families about hospice?
- How do I tell the patient's family that death is imminent? What should I say to notify the family that the patient has died?
- Can I discuss organ and tissue donation with the family?
- Who discusses autopsy with the family?

WHAT ARE THE MOST COMMON NEEDS OF THE TERMINALLY ILL PATIENT?

The easiest way to identify a patient's needs is to ask. However, an open-ended question such as, "Do you need anything?" may not yield a comprehensive response from the patient. The nurse may elicit a better response by pulling up a chair and acknowledging the recent diagnosis or by suggesting interventions that are possible or available.

How to Say It

"I know you've had some bad news about your diagnosis. I want to be sure that we take care of all your needs while you are in the hospital and when you go home. Can you tell me how we can help you?"

"Other patients that I've cared for under your circumstances have wanted ___, ___, and ___. Will any of these be helpful to you?"

A large study of terminally ill patients' needs was done. Patients from six geographic areas of the United States who had an expected survival of less than 6 months were surveyed. The analysis identified eight factors that represent what terminally ill patients care about[1] (Table 3-1).

Table 3-1 Factors Important to Terminally Ill Patients and Nursing Interventions

Factors[1]	Nursing Interventions
Patient-Clinician relationship	Assignment continuity Time spent just talking and listening
Social connectedness	Open visiting, including children Chaplain visits
Caregiving needs	Symptom control Assistance with ADLs Home care referral at discharge Hospice referral at discharge
Psychological distress	Time spent listening Mental health consult Anxiolytics
Spirituality/religiousness	Spiritual history Respect rituals and traditions Chaplain visits
Personal acceptance	Assignment continuity Open visiting Chaplain visits
Sense of purpose	Assignment continuity Time spent listening Open visiting Chaplain visits
Clinician communication	Clear, honest communication Avoid jargon, acronyms, medical terminology Frequent updates

Caregiving needs may need to be addressed first. A patient with uncontrolled symptoms and/or an inability to complete activities of daily living (ADLs) will be unprepared to attend to the other needs listed in Table 3-1. Strategies to assess and treat common symptoms are discussed in Chapter 4.

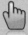

Clinical Alert

Uncontrolled symptoms will hinder patients from attending to their psychological, social, and spiritual needs.

HOW SHOULD NURSES ADDRESS PATIENT NEEDS FOR SOCIAL CONNECTEDNESS, PSYCHOLOGICAL DISTRESS, SPIRITUALITY, AND PATIENT-NURSE RELATIONSHIP?

Nurses spend more time at patient's bedside than any other discipline in the hospital. This gives the nurse a high amount of visibility and access to the patient to ascertain and address **patient needs for social connectedness, psychological distress, and spirituality.** Nurses also sit on hospital committees and task forces and are able to represent the patient's perspective when policies are written or revised.

Patient-Nurse Relationship

Often in hospitals today it is difficult for the patient to have a primary nurse because of flexible scheduling. The terminally ill patient values a clinician relationship and paradoxically some nurses avoid the terminally ill patient because of fear of saying or doing the wrong thing. Additionally, the nursing shortage has left many hospital units short-handed and it may be difficult to find time to just sit with the patient to talk and listen.

Perhaps during change of shift report nurses can plan for the terminally ill patient's nurse to have some 1:1 time with the patient. Alternatively, the assigned nurse can try to mix talking and listening with care delivery such as during assessment or when passing medications or changing dressings. Additionally, the night nurse may find more time to sit with the sleepless patient and listen to his or her concerns. As often as scheduling permits the patient should be assigned the same nurse.

Social Connectedness

As patients approach the end of their lives relationships become more important. For some, there is a need to reconnect if estranged, seek or grant forgiveness, or make restitution. This is an even more important need if the patient is actively dying while in the hospital. Opportunities for social exchange are becoming limited while the need to "be with" becomes stronger. This is not the time for restrictions on visitation.

Most hospitals impose some limitation on visitors to patients in order to control traffic flow, afford time for patient rest or sleep, and provide privacy such as during physician rounds. However, there are always exceptions to visitor policies and the nurse is usually the gatekeeper with the most control over when to allow exceptions to the policy. Dying patients should have unrestricted access to the people who are important to them, including children.

Unrestricted visits can best be accommodated if the patient is in or is moved to a private room. A hospital mechanism for communicating the policy exception is also helpful so the patient or family does not need to repeat the request every day or every shift. This may take the form of an order in the chart, an entry in the patient kardex, a notation in the electronic medical record, or a list kept at the desk where visitors get their passes.

When the patient is near death one or more family members may stay continuously at the bedside; this is sometimes referred to as a "death vigil." For many, it is important to be with the patient at the moment of death. Nurses can accommodate this need by moving extra chairs, ideally one or more recliners, into the patient room. Fresh ice water, cups, juice, and tissues are useful and when placed in the room provide evidence of nurse caring.

Other patients' visitors may ask why they have to go home in the evening when they see visitors staying around the clock. A reply that doesn't breach the dying patient's confidentiality is something like this: "The patient in that room has special circumstances that mean the family must stay close. Your loved one doesn't have those special circumstances." Usually, visitors of other patients have an idea about why the dying patient has open visiting.

Sadly, some patients have no family or friends. This lack of social connectedness may be preferred by the patient or be the result of an unfortunate circumstance. Volunteers, sitters, the nursing staff, and the hospital chaplain are all sources of social support for the patient who is alone.

Clinical Alert
Hospital policies may impose barriers to meeting the needs of the terminally ill patient. Policies can be changed.

Psychological Distress

A patient has psychological distress when he or she reports any depression, anxiety, difficulty sleeping, fear of going to sleep, bad dreams, night terrors, and fear of death. The nurse can be responsive to the patient's psychological distress by listening, showing compassion, and acknowledging the patient's emotions. The patient with psychological distress may fear being alone and will ring the call bell frequently. Frequent, even brief, interactions between the nurse and patient may be helpful. Moving the patient to a room where there is more traffic may also be useful.

How to Say It

"Sometimes patients with your condition experience fear or anxiety or sadness. Are you feeling sad or fearful or anxious? Do you want to tell me about how you are feeling?"

"How are you sleeping?"

"Are you afraid to sleep?"

"What frightens you about going to sleep? Are you afraid you might die?"

"Shall I sit with you until you fall asleep?"

Patients with psychological distress may benefit from consultation with a psychiatrist, psychologist, psychiatric nurse practitioner, or life stress counselor, if available. Some patients receive benefit from treatment with antidepressants or anxiolytics. (See Chapter 4.)

Spirituality and Religiousness

One definition of spirituality is "a unifying force of a person, the essence of being that permeates all of life and is manifested in one's being, knowing, and doing; the interconnectedness with self, others, nature, and God/Life force/Absolute/Transcendent."[2] Religion is understood to be the organized, codified, or institutionalized beliefs and practices that characterize one's spirituality. The patient is likely to have personal definitions of both spirituality and religion. (See Appendix H.)

A spiritual assessment is a means of determining what the patient's needs are, and awareness of spirituality often increases when the patient learns about terminal illness. One model for spiritual assessment uses the acronym FICA as given below.[3] Documentation of the patient's responses ensures communication across caregivers.

How to Say It	
F (Faith)	Do you have a faith belief? What is it that gives your life meaning?
I (Import or influence)	What importance does your faith have in your life? How does your faith belief influence your life?
C (Community)	Are you a member of a faith community? How does this support you?
A (Address)	How would you like me to address these issues in your care?

Puchalski has recommended the following spiritual care interventions:[4]

- Listening to the concerns, feelings, and beliefs of the patient
- Providing a safe environment and an attentive ear so that the patient can express feelings and experiences associated with illness, stress, and dying
- Providing opportunities for the patient to express grief, anger, despair, sorrow, happiness, joy, and confusion
- Suggesting important relationships that might help the patient (family, clergy, counselors)
- Referring to professional spiritual care providers (chaplains)
- Spiritual practice such as yoga or meditation
- Rituals, sacraments
- Worship or other spiritual services
- Prayer
- Sacred reading (Bible, Koran, Torah)
- Reflective readings from poetry or literature
- Journaling by patient or family

Sometimes patients or their families ask the nurse to pray with them. The nurse should view this intimacy as a sign of respect and inclusion of the nurse into a special family moment. Rejecting this invitation could be hurtful to the patient. Accepting the invitation graciously and standing quietly with the family may be an option. The nurse should seek support from the hospital chaplain if the family asks for someone to lead a prayer since that is a specialized skill.

WHAT ARE THE MOST COMMON NEEDS OF THE TERMINALLY ILL PATIENT'S FAMILY?

An early study identified two categories of spousal needs when the patient is dying in the hospital: relationship with the patient, and family needs for communication and support.[5] Relationship with the patient included the need to be with the patient, to feel helpful to that person, and to be assured that the patient is comfortable. The nurse, as previously stated, is the gatekeeper to the patient. The nurse can meet family needs by permitting unrestricted visitation, allowing family to help with basic care, and provide assurances about the patient's comfort.

Families also have strong communication needs. Anticipatory grief, grief and bereavement needs of families are presented in Chapter 6.

Joan Bright, RN, is caring for a patient, Mrs. Peabody, who has suffered an acute ischemic stroke. In spite of medical treatment the patient is declining and not expected to survive. Joan sits in on the meeting with the patient's family when the primary physician explains the diagnosis, prognosis, and treatment goals. The physician tells them the patient has had "an acute left MCA infarct" complicated by "worsening cerebral edema." He goes on to tell them "her prognosis is poor" and "we need to know what you want us to do." The family listens politely and after the physician leaves they turn to Joan and ask, "What was he trying to tell us?"

WHAT IS THE NURSE'S ROLE IN COMMUNICATING WITH PATIENT OR FAMILY ABOUT THE PATIENT'S TERMINAL ILLNESS?

As discussed in Chapter 1, communication with the patient and family is a standard of professional nursing practice.[6] Successful nursing communication is characterized by collaboration with the patient's physician, listening as much as speaking, and acknowledging patient or family emotions. The nurse is also expected to inform the patient's physician about any gaps in communication.

Joan explains the diagnosis to the patient's family using plain, simple English by saying, "Mrs. Peobody has had a stroke from a blockage in the circulation to her brain. This means that a part of her brain is no longer functioning. Additionally, there is swelling around the brain from the shock of the stroke and Mrs. Peabody is not improving, in fact, the doctor was telling you that Mrs. Peabody might die." As expected, the family displays grief behaviors and Joan leaves them momentarily to call the physician. When he responds she tells him that the family did not understand his previous discussion but that she has clarified the intended message. She asks him to return to continue discussion with the family and lets the family know what time to expect the follow-up discussion.

Few physicians and nurses in current practice have been taught how to break bad news. Reliance on medical terminology, acronyms, and jargon leaves the family confused. Additionally, patients and families are often intimidated by their loss of control in the health-care setting and may be shy about acknowledging their lack of understanding.

WHAT ARE THE COMMUNICATION NEEDS OF THE DYING PATIENT'S FAMILY?

In an early study of the needs of critically ill patients' families, 5 of the 10 most important needs were for communication:[7]

- To be called at home about changes in the condition of the patient
- To know the prognosis
- To have questions answered honestly
- To receive information about the patient once a day
- To have explanations given in terms that are understandable

In a study of the needs of spouses of patients dying in the hospital these additional communication needs were identified:[5]

- Assurance of the comfort of the patient
- Information about the patient's condition
- Informed about the impending death

Ineffective communication about dying is frequently cited as a barrier to optimal care at the end of life.[8] Nurses have the skills and the opportunity to bridge communication gaps because of their frequent contact with the patient and family and the trust that patients and families have in nurses.

HOW SHOULD BAD NEWS BE BROKEN?

The following steps and considerations make this process effective and compassionate regardless of who is breaking the bad news.

Prepare in Advance

Who is going to lead the discussion with the patient or family? Where will the discussion take place?

The bedside is best if the patient is participating, a private area with adequate seating for all is preferred if the patient is not participating. Patients who are alert and have decision-making capacity should participate if they want. Occasionally, a patient will defer decisionmaking to family. Assuring privacy for the patient in a semiprivate room or ward is challenging. Removing the patient, if able, or the roommates for the duration of the discussion is ideal. Barring that option, the team will need to lower their voices to assure confidentiality.

Who needs to be present?

The primary physician or designee, assigned staff nurse, and other relevant clinical team members or consultants should be present if possible. Support personnel such as social workers or chaplains may also be helpful.

When should the discussion occur?

Timing is important to consider so all personnel and the patient's family can be present. Choosing a time when interruptions of the clinical staff can be avoided is also important.

Establish a Therapeutic Milieu

As mentioned, privacy at the patient's bedside may be difficult to achieve. A private space, with enough chairs for all involved is important wherever the discussion occurs. A classroom, conference room, or family waiting area can be appropriated for this purpose. A sign on the door stating, "Family meeting in progress" will minimize interruptions.

Everyone should be seated, including the clinical personnel. This establishes eye contact and avoids psychological barriers.

Before discussing the patient's condition it is important to introduce everyone to the patient and/or family and to identify who is present for the patient.

Ascertain What Is Known and Introduce the Goal

Ask the patient and/or family about what is known. Listen carefully to the responses as this will indicate the patient or family literacy about the illness or any misconceptions.

Introduce the goal of honest, direct communication. Nearly all patients or families want this direct approach and will acknowledge this.

How to Say It

"What do you know about your condition? (or 'What do you know about the patient's condition?') We want to add to what you already know."

"It is our custom to be honest and straightforward even when we are communicating bad news."

Communicate Diagnosis and Prognosis

Using plain, simple English tell the patient and/or family the diagnosis without using jargon, acronyms, or medical terminology. Ask if the explanation has been understood. Clarify misconceptions or confusion. Avoid overemphasis on the medical diagnostics, get to the point. Some of our common terms in health care are used in a different way in simple English and can lead to confusion (Box 3-1).

Box 3-1 Confusing Terms

Medical Usage	Common Usage
A negative CT scan is normal	Negative is pessimistic
Positive HIV results are abnormal	Positive is optimistic
Illness is progressing (getting worse)	Progress suggests improvement

When English is not the first spoken language of the patient or family it may be useful to bring in an interpreter. Most hospitals have a policy about interpreters in response to a Joint Commission on Accreditation of Healthcare Organizations (JCAHO) standard.

The prognosis should also be explained in direct language. Terms such as *prognosis* are not commonly used by lay people. Say *dying* or *death* if that is the intended message; other euphemisms such as *declining* and *taking a turn for the worse* are not clear enough and their use will be a barrier to planning the dying patient's care. Furthermore, if the family is not told clearly that the patient is dying they may miss opportunities for closure and be unnecessarily surprised when the patient dies. The nurse can show empathy by describing how breaking the news makes him or her feel.

How to Say It

"I'm sorry to tell you that this illness has no cure. It will get worse over time and someday he will die from this."

"This type of stroke is nearly always fatal. That means most people who have this type of stroke die from it."

"This is a progressive illness that has no cure. That means it will keep getting worse over time. Our tests show that it has reached the terminal stage."

"I'm very sad to have to tell you that his condition is worsening and we believe he will die soon."

"I regret that there are no further treatments that will improve her condition. In fact, she shows signs that she will die soon."

Throughout this communication the person delivering the news must pause often to let the patient or family speak or ask questions, to acknowledge emotions, and to ascertain understanding.

HOW SHOULD TREATMENT GOALS AND DNR BE DISCUSSED?

After the diagnosis and prognosis have been discussed, the patient and/or family should be asked if they are ready to proceed into a discussion of treatment options. Some will need a break to absorb the news particularly if it was unexpected.

How to Say It

"I know we've given you a lot of difficult information. We want to talk about care options with you. Do you need some time to absorb the news?"

"Are you able to let me discuss care options now or do you need a break to absorb all this information?"

The point of the discussion is to clarify treatment goals, not "get the code status." While it is important to know if an attempt at resuscitation should be made at the time of patient death, it is equally important to know how to care for the patient prior to death, with or without resuscitation. Hence, the discussion should center on goals and when the goals are clarified the pertinent interventions become clear. Some clinicians offer the patient or family a list of interventions and ask them to choose. This is an illogical, backward approach because an intervention may not be useful in the context of some goals.

Goals can be categorized as *cure*, *rehabilitation*, *prolongation*, and *palliation*. The following vignettes illustrate discussion of goals.

Mrs. Peabody's family meets again with the physician and the nurse, Joan, to discuss treatment goals after Joan has clarified the diagnosis and prognosis. The physician repeats his earlier question, "What do you want us to do?" Joan interrupts to say, "Perhaps you can tell this family what the options are" and the family nods. The physician tells the family that prolongative treatment is possible, but will not improve the brain damage from the stroke and a palliative care approach is the alternative. He answers the family's questions with Joan's assistance and a mutual agreement to focus on palliation is achieved. His earlier open-ended question was not useful because the family was inexperienced and did not know the options.

Erma Brown is an 89-year-old woman living independently in her own home. She is a widow and her adult children live nearby and check on her daily. She is proud of her independence. On one of her daily checks, Mrs. Brown's daughter finds her mother on the floor, crying from pain and she has been incontinent of urine.

At the hospital, the initial workup reveals a left hip fracture and the orthopedic surgeons believe she is a good candidate for hip replacement since she was previously ambulatory and self-sufficient. Treatment goals are not discussed but cure and rehabilitation of the acute insult is the default plan of care.

Mrs. Brown's postoperative course is complicated by pneumonia and she declines rapidly. A meeting with her family is convened and treatment goals are discussed. Mrs. Brown's children report that their mother values independence and is not afraid to die. They also report her previously stated wish for no aggressive therapy if her health failed. Thus, a mutual agreement is achieved to change the treatment goal to palliation. Once the goal is established, the clinicians can prescribe interventions that correspond to the goal and the patient's needs and thus, running through a list of interventions with the family is unnecessary. Mrs. Brown's family can be told by the clinicians which interventions will be continued and why and which are nonbeneficial or painful procedures that *will be discontinued, such as physical therapy, labs, x-rays, and antibiotics.*

Andrew Bocci *is a 19-year-old college student admitted after a motor vehicle accident in which he sustained blunt trauma mostly involving the chest. He has numerous bilateral rib fractures, bilateral hemopneumothoraces, and respiratory failure requiring mechanical ventilation. Since his prognosis is indeterminate at admission there is no discussion of goals, in fact, cure is the default expectation and all necessary interventions, including resuscitation will be employed.*

After a week of ICU care, Andrew has declined. He has refractory adult respiratory distress syndrome and is oxygenating poorly in spite of mechanical ventilation and 100% oxygen. Additionally, he is in septic shock with Dopamine and Levophed infusing at maximal therapeutic rates. Finally, he is in anuric renal failure. With multiple organ system failure the prognosis is nearly 100% and a goal clarification meeting with Andrew's family is planned.

The surgeons explain the diagnosis and high probability of imminent death to Andrew's family. They also explain the nonbenefit of resuscitation in this clinical context. After answering all questions, the surgeons and family reach an agreement to change treatment goals from the default "cure" to palliation and to withdraw life-sustaining measures. The relevant interventions flow from this goal such as ceasing labs, x-rays, nonbeneficial lines, tubes, and catheters. Withdrawal of fluids, pressors, and the ventilator are planned.

Families benefit from a recommendation about one or more alternative goals. Asking a family to tell us what to do puts a burden on the family who may not have the health-care knowledge needed to make a decision. Similarly, asking a family if they want CPR without making a recommendation can lead to a decision to attempt CPR even when it is not expected to be useful. Finally, asking a family to choose the interventions is relegating clinical decision making (Table 3-2).

Table 3-2 Discussing Treatment Goals and Resuscitation

Wrong approach	Correct approach	Rationale
If your mother's heart stops do you want us to use CPR to restart it?	When a patient in your mother's condition reaches the end of life, aggressive measures like CPR are not effective and can cause distress. We recommend no attempts at resuscitation if she dies in spite of our treatment.	The *wrong* approach implies that CPR will be successful. The *wrong* approach provides no clinical context or recommendation to the family.
We have a list of possible treatments for you to decide about for your father. Do you want: • CPR • Intubation • Feeding tube • Antibiotics • Blood transfusions • Dialysis • Fries (smile)	Your father has a terminal illness and we don't have a treatment that will improve his condition, however, there are a number of things we can do to relieve his pain or other distress and help him and your family prepare for his death. We recommend that all his treatment focuses on palliation, in other words comfort and emotional and family support.	The *wrong* approach has no associated clinical context or treatment goal. The *wrong* approach could lead to an illogical plan such as CPR but no intubation. The *wrong* approach implies that one, some, or all these interventions will be beneficial. The *wrong* approach gives clinical decision making to the family. The *correct* approach shares a decision with family about the goal of treatment after an explanation of diagnosis, prognosis, and benefit of the recommended goal. The *correct* approach emphasizes what can be done for the patient and family.

HOW DO THESE DISCUSSIONS OCCUR WHEN THE PATIENT HAS A DYSFUNCTIONAL FAMILY?

A dysfunctional family is characterized by being unable to function as a family unit and/or being estranged from one another. Often chemical abuse or mental illness in one or more family members is a contributing factor.

The following are dysfunctional family behaviors:

* Focus on negative feelings and relationships
  — *"My sister never helps with our mother's care."*
* Focus on fault finding
  — *"Why doesn't anyone ever turn our father?"*
  — *"He didn't have any bedsores when he was admitted."*
* Display exaggerated response to events often with raised voices
  — *"What you mean we have to learn to give him insulin? How do you expect us to learn something like that?"*
* Reluctant to agree with other family members or health-care team
  — *"My brother is wrong, he doesn't understand our mother the way I do"*
* Uncomfortable with each other, seek individual meetings with physician
* Need a great deal of attention, regardless of staff's other demands

The heightened emotions that accompany terminal illness often exacerbate preexisting family dysfunction. Family conferences may be compromised since the family lacks cohesion and may be more accustomed to fighting than reaching consensus. It may be best to have single conferences with individuals and seek agreement individually about the treatment plan. This will take more time but a group family meeting to obtain consensus may prove to be an exercise in futility.

When dysfunctional family behavior becomes disruptive it is important to

- Set limits, politely.
- Identify expected, mutually respectful behaviors.
- Identify frequency of communication, number of contacts, time of day.
- Use a consistent approach across shifts and among staff.

How to Say It

"I can see that your family doesn't always get along. It's important for us to maintain a quiet environment for all our patients. I have to ask you to save your arguments for when you leave the hospital, or if you can't wait, please keep your voices soft."

"It's clear to us that your family has special needs. We will do our best to accommodate everyone, but we have some expectations. Everyone in the family will get a chance to speak, but we need a chance to talk as well. We will not raise our voices or interrupt or be critical when we talk to you; we ask you to do the same when you speak with us."

"We want your family to have regular updates but there isn't enough time in the day for us to have a long discussion with everyone individually. The nurse responsible for your loved one's care will be available at x time every day for 20 minutes to give an update." (Choose a mutually agreeable time and stick with it.)

WHAT NEEDS TO HAPPEN IF THERE IS NO MUTUAL AGREEMENT ABOUT TREATMENT GOALS?

When the patient or surrogates and health-care team remain conflicted about treatment goals there are several options to reach consensus.

First, has the communication been effective?

Faulty communication is the reason for most cases of disagreement. Do all parties to the discussion and decision have the same understanding of the patient's diagnosis, prognosis, and goal options? Has the family had enough time to absorb the bad news before being asked to make decisions about recommendations? What barriers to communication or misconceptions have been overlooked? Review the previous communications and ascertain if the process could be improved. Bring in a consultant, such as palliative care, to assist with further discussions. Alternatively, social workers and chaplains are skillful at resolving communication gaps.

Second, is the difference of opinion about nonbeneficial treatment?

Was nonbeneficial treatment offered as if it would be of benefit? For example, was the family asked if CPR should be done without any discussion of its nonbenefit in terminal illness. In other words, did someone say, "If the patient's heart stops do you want us to restart it with CPR?" without describing the illness, prognosis, and without making a recommendation to refrain from CPR? Does the hospital have a policy about resolving demands for nonbeneficial treatment if they cannot be resolved with effective communication? A consult to the Hospital Ethics Committee may address this issue.

Third, is the barrier identifying the most valid surrogate?

Are the potential surrogates in dispute about who should make decisions? In some states the law directs who should serve as surrogate when the patient has lost decision-making capacity. Hospital policy about consent and surrogacy may also outline a process. Additionally, social workers or chaplains can be helpful in this type of case.

The ultimate goal is to reach consensus among all parties and this may take time and patience.

WHAT CAN I TELL PATIENTS AND THEIR FAMILIES ABOUT HOSPICE?

Hospice is both a philosophy of care and a model for care delivery. When a hospice referral is recommended to a patient and/or family questions about hospice may arise. Families need to know:

- Hospice care is covered by most insurances and Medicare and often Medicaid
- Hospice care is provided in many settings, including the patient's home, long-term care facilities, inpatient units (if patient meets criteria), and free-standing hospice facilities (not available in all communities)
- Hospice care emphasizes symptom management and psycho-emotional-spiritual care
- Hospice care provides support to families before and after the patient's death

Some hospitals have a hospice coordinator or liaison on staff who can counsel families about hospice. Alternatively, the hospice the patient is being referred to will send personnel to meet with the family and answer questions, if needed. (See Appendix I.)

HOW DO I TELL THE PATIENT'S FAMILY THAT DEATH IS IMMINENT? WHAT SHOULD I SAY TO NOTIFY THE FAMILY THAT THE PATIENT HAS DIED?

Families often ask the nurse to estimate how long the patient has to live. This is a complicated question and collaboration with the physician to provide a response is essential. A precise estimation is not possible; conversely overestimating is not helpful because the patient and family may not achieve life-closure tasks if we are not honest about time remaining, particularly if out-of-town family needs to travel. Suggesting a range of time that is consistent with the patient's functional status may be best. Conferring with experts in terminal illness prognostication to answer this family question may be helpful.

How to Say It

"We can't know the exact amount of time left with certainty, but with other patients who have reached this stage death usually occurred in (minutes to hours) or (hours to a day or two) or (days to weeks) or (weeks to months)."

When a patient's death is *expected,* families want to know when death is imminent, especially if the family is not at the hospital. They may want to return to be with the patient. A clear communication is essential. Don't tell the family they must come in; some family members may prefer not to witness the patient's death.

When the patient has died the communication should also be direct. Sometimes families will have preferences about who to call and whether to break the news over the phone. These needs can be elicited in advance and noted in the record.

How to Say It

"Hello, Mrs. Tompkins. I'm _____ and I'm caring for your husband this evening. I'm calling to tell you that his condition is changing and I believe he may die soon. I've placed some extra chairs in his room in case you or other family members want to come to the hospital. Please drive slowly and carefully if you decide to come in."

"Mr. Wilkinson, I'm _____ and I've been caring for your wife tonight. I'm calling with sad news (pause); your wife died a short time ago. (Allow time for initial reaction, sometimes weeping.) I'll be here to assist you if you want to come see her. Please have someone in your family drive you while your emotions are intense."

When a patient's death is *unexpected,* but imminent, a critical notification to the family is best.[9] This type of phrasing would also be appropriate if the patient has died and the death notification would occur in person when the family comes to the hospital.

How to Say It

"Hello, Mr. Zabor. I'm _____ and I'm caring for your sister today. She has had a sudden, unexpected change in her condition. We need to talk with you and the rest of her family. Will you come to the hospital?"

The family might ask if the patient has died. The response is "yes" (allow time for reaction), encourage safe driving to the hospital to have all questions answered.

CAN I DISCUSS ORGAN AND TISSUE DONATION WITH THE FAMILY?

NO. The Center for Medicare and Medicaid Services (CMS) guidelines require that a designated requestor discusses organ and tissue donation. Most hospitals rely on personnel from the organ procurement organization in their state. (See Appendix K.)

WHO DISCUSSES AUTOPSY WITH THE FAMILY?

Elective autopsies are encouraged in teaching facilities. Generally, the physician who is responsible for the patient's care or the physician who pronounces death offers autopsy to the family. When the patient has died secondary to trauma, homicide, suicide, or from unknown causes the death is reported to the county coroner or medical examiner. It is the legal purview of the medical examiner to require an autopsy. The nurse or physician can explain this to the family.

CLOSING VIGNETTE

Mr. and Mrs. Mitchell are shocked and frightened about the patient's poor prognosis and probable limited survival. Mr. Mitchell sits by the bed and cries, while Mrs. Mitchell struggles to soothe him while being upset herself. The nurse closes the door, sits down, and asks "What can I do to help you both? I can see how upset you are and while I don't know what you are experiencing, I can imagine how badly you feel." Mr. Mitchell says, "There's nothing you can do, unless you have a cure for cancer up your sleeve." Mrs. Mitchell says, "I don't want to be alone right now, can my husband stay a bit later? I know visiting hours end soon." The nurse assures them that Mr. Mitchell can stay. She gets him a special pass to show security when he moves around the hospital. She also moves a special bed-chair into the room that will allow Mr. Mitchell to stretch out and sleep if he stays all night. The nurse indicates that she will have some open time later in the shift and will come sit with them to answer questions and learn more about their needs.

CLOSING PEARLS

Nurses have a great deal of independent authority to meet patient and family needs at the end of life. The patient's needs for social connectedness, spiritual, and psychological support are met by the nurse through providing unrestricted visiting, conducting a spiritual history, being with and listening to the patient, and consulting other disciplines such as the chaplain.

The best antidote for families' uncertainty is effective communication.[10] Nurses are ideally suited to meet a family's communication needs.

REFERENCES

1. Emanuel LL, Alpert HR, Baldwin DC, Emanuel EJ. What terminally ill patients care about: toward a validated construct of patients' perspectives. *J Palliat Med.* 2000;3(4):419–431.

2. Dossey BM, Guzzetta CE. Holistic nursing practice. In: Dossey BM, Guzzetta CE, eds. *Holistic nursing: A handbook for practice.* 3rd ed. Rockville, MD: Aspen; 2000:5–26.

3. Puchalski CM. Taking a spiritual history: FICA. *Spirituality and medicine connections.* 1999;3:1.

4. Puchalski CM. Spirituality in health: the role of spirituality in critical care. *Crit Care Clin.* 2004;20:487–504.

5. Hampe SO. Needs of the grieving spouse in a hospital setting. *Nurs Res.* 1975;24:113–120.

6. American Nurses Association. *Scope and standards of practice* Washington, D.C.: American Nurses Association; 2004.

7. Molter NC. Needs of relatives of critically ill patients: a descriptive study. *Heart & Lung.* 1979;8:332–339.

8. Field MJ, Cassel CK, eds. *Approaching death: Improving care at the end of life.* Washington, D.C.: National Academy Press; 1997.

9. Viswanathan R, Clark JJ, Viswanathan K. Physicians' and the public's attitudes on communication about death. *Arch Intern Med.* 1986;146:2029–2033.

10. Kirchhoff KT, Walker L, Hutton A, Spuhler V, Cole BV, Clemmer T. The vortex: families' experiences with death in the intensive care unit. *Am J Crit Care.* May 2002;11(3):200–209.

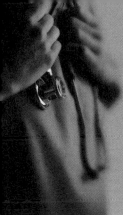

Chapter 4

CARE OF THE PATIENT BEFORE AND AFTER DEATH

Meg Whitney, APN, is the palliative care nurse practitioner. She provides consultation in the hospital and directs the care of patients on the Palliative Care Unit (PCU). Currently, there are eight patients on the PCU. Some patients are on the unit for aggressive symptom management before returning home, others are actively dying and will stay on the unit until death (Table 4-1).

❓ Frequently Asked Questions

- What are the most common symptoms experienced by patients nearing the end of life?
- What are the best methods for symptom assessment?
- How should symptoms be assessed if the patient cannot self-report?
- What can be done to relieve symptoms with medications and besides medication?
- Will patients become addicted if they take opioids?
- How do we give opioids to the patient who is a substance abuser?
- Will opioids hasten death?
- What can be done if the patient's symptoms are refractory to treatment?

Table 4-1 Unit Census with Patient Age, Name, Diagnosis

Age	Name	Diagnosis
83	Wilbur	Alzheimer disease, pneumonia
62	Frances	COPD
28	Celeste	Hypoglycemic coma
48	Thomas	Colon cancer, bowel obstruction
59	Susan	Ovarian cancer
81	Clarence	Hemorrhagic stroke
63	Elaine	Cirrhosis
78	John	Heart failure

- When can the patient be an organ or tissue donor?
- Who can pronounce the patient's death?
- Who notifies the family about the death? Can a nurse do this?
- How should the family be notified? What should be said or not said?
- Should the family be notified by phone if they are not present?
- When is the death reported to a medical examiner or coroner?
- How should the body be prepared for family viewing?
- How long can the body and the family remain in the room?

WHAT ARE THE MOST COMMON SYMPTOMS EXPERIENCED BY PATIENTS NEARING THE END OF LIFE?

The most common symptoms experienced by patients with terminal illness are outlined in Table 4-2. Retained upper airway secretions are also commonly experienced by patients when they are near death but the prevalence has not been previously measured.

Table 4-2 Symptom Prevalence Across Common Terminal Illnesses[1]

Symptoms	Cancer (percent)	AIDS (percent)	Heart disease (percent)	COPD (percent)	Renal disease (percent)
Pain	35–96	63–80	41–77	34–77	47–50
Confusion	6–93	30–5	18–32	18–33	—
Dyspnea	10–70	11–62	60–88	90–95	11–62
Nausea	6–68	43–49	17–48	—	30–43
Constipation	23–65	34–35	38–42	27–44	29–70
Diarrhea	3–29	30–90	12	—	21
Anorexia	30–92	51	21–41	35–67	25–64

WHAT ARE THE BEST METHODS FOR SYMPTOM ASSESSMENT? HOW SHOULD SYMPTOMS BE ASSESSED IF THE PATIENT CANNOT SELF-REPORT?

The most reliable way to assess patient symptoms and any associated distress is by asking the patient to identify if any symptoms are present. For each symptom identified a multidimensional assessment is helpful to know. A patient may have a symptom but no distress. When a symptom is identified, such as breathlessness, the nurse should inquire about:

- Intensity/severity
- Quality (e.g., describe the symptom)
- Duration (e.g., continuous or episodic)
- Triggers (e.g., activity)
- What brings relief?

Patients who are near death may be confused or have cognitive impairment such that it is difficult or impossible to elicit a symptom self-report. Behavioral assessment may guide the nurse's assessment; alternatively the patient's family may be able to offer insights into the patient's comfort versus distress.

Clinical Alert
An attempt to elicit a patient self-report about symptoms and symptom distress should precede reliance on behaviors or family opinion.

Pain Assessment

Pain is an unpleasant sensory or emotional experience associated with actual or potential tissue damage or described in terms of such damage.[2] In the hospital, pain is assessed at admission, every time vital signs are measured, and after analgesia administration. Common assessment methods include:

- Numeric rating scale—ranges from 0 to 10 with 0 signifying no pain, and 10 signifying the most severe pain. Patient reports are trended in the nursing documentation. It is generally understood that scores from 1 to 3 suggest mild pain, 4 to 6 indicates moderate pain, and 7 to 10 implies severe pain.

- Visual analog scale (VAS)—a horizontal line, usually anchored at 0 and 10. Patient points to a place on the line that represents pain intensity.

- Wong-Baker FACES scale—a tool developed for use with children, although some institutions use it with adults[3] (Figure 4-1).

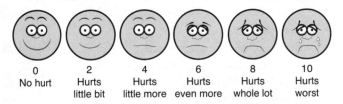

| 0 | 2 | 4 | 6 | 8 | 10 |
| No hurt | Hurts little bit | Hurts little more | Hurts even more | Hurts whole lot | Hurts worst |

Figure 4-1   Wong-Baker FACES scale. (From Hockenberry MJ, Wilson D, Winkelstein ML: Wong's Essentials of Pediatric Nursing, ed. 7, St. Louis, 2005, p. 1259. Used with permission. Copyright, Mosby.)

- Yes or no inquiry—sick patients may be unable to use any of the aforedescribed scales. The simplest way to elicit a patient self-report about pain experienced is to ask, "Are you having pain?"
- Behaviors—grimacing, rigidity, wincing, shutting of eyes, verbalization, moaning, and clenching of fists.[4]

Dyspnea Assessment

Dyspnea is a subjective experience of breathing discomfort that consists of qualitatively distinct sensations that vary in intensity.[5] Patients may use synonymous terms such as *short of breath* or *breathlessness*. Patients at risk for dyspnea (see Table 4-2) should be assessed with the same frequency as pain assessment. Common assessment methods follow:

- Numeric rating scale—ranges from 0 to 10 with 0 signifying no breathlessness, and 10 signifying the most severe breathlessness. Patient reports are trended in the nursing documentation.
- Dyspnea VAS—a 100-mm line anchored at 0 indicating no breathlessness, and 100 signifying the worst possible breathlessness with tick marks every 10 mm. A vertical line was preferred by patients in one study [6] (Figure 4-2).
- Yes or No inquiry—sick patients may be unable to use any of the aforedescribed scales. The simplest way to elicit a patient self-report about dyspnea experienced is to ask, "Are you short of breath?"
- Behaviors—tachypnea (respiratory rate >baseline), tachycardia, accessory muscle use (elevation of the clavicle on inspiration), fearful facial expression (Figure 4-3), paradoxical breathing (inward movement of the abdomen on inspiration), grunting at end-expiration, and nasal flaring.[7–9]

Nausea/Vomiting/Diarrhea Assessment

Nausea is a feeling of sickness with an urge to vomit. While nausea can only be assessed from the patient's report, vomiting

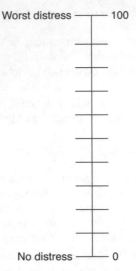

Worst distress ——— 100

No distress ——— 0

Figure 4-2   Sample dyspnea visual analog scale (not illustrated to scale).

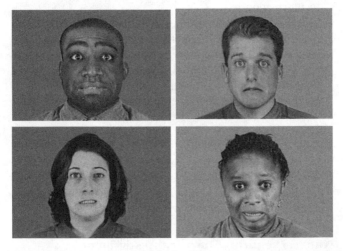

Figure 4-3   Examples of fearful facial expression. Reproduced, with permission, Ursula Hess, PhD, University of Montreal, Montreal, Quebec, Canada.

and diarrhea are visible symptoms. Documenting the frequency of episodes of vomiting and/or diarrhea should be done. Additionally, the presence of fecal material in emesis and the presence of blood in either emesis or diarrhea should be noted and reported to the prescriber caring for the patient.

Constipation Assessment

Constipation is infrequent (and frequently incomplete) bowel movements. The frequency and consistency of bowel movements constitutes constipation assessment. Opioid medications, decreased fluid intake, and decreased mobility increase the patient's risk of becoming constipated. Generally, a patient should experience a daily bowel movement if he or she is still eating or receiving enteral nourishment.

Anorexia Assessment

Anorexia is a loss of appetite or an aversion to food. Loss of appetite is common in terminal illnesses and often is the herald of the active dying phase. Collaboration with a clinical dietician is a useful way to assess anorexia, its triggers, and possible interventions. When the patient is not actively dying it may be useful to collect a diet diary and elicit food preferences and food aversions from the patient or family.

Delirium Assessment

Delirium is an acute and relatively sudden decline in attention focus, perception, and cognition. It is common in terminally ill patients and during the active dying phase.[11] The patient may display one or more of the following signs:

- Rapid change in level of consciousness
- Acute onset, usually in hours or days
- Inability to focus or a change in attention
- Disorientation
- Disturbance in sleep-wake cycle
- Fluctuation over the course of the day, often worsening at night

• Hyperalert agitation
• Delusions or hallucinations

Retained Upper Airway Secretions

Noisy, gurgling respirations signify retained upper airway secretions. This is familiarly referred to as "rattling" or "death rattle." It occurs commonly in the patient's last hours as a consequence of decreasing consciousness with decreased cough and/or swallow.

Comprehensive symptom assessment tools that trend multiple symptoms simultaneously and over time are available. See the Edmonton Symptom Assessment Scale (Appendix L) and the Memorial Symptom Scale (Appendix M) for examples.

Wilbur is in the advanced stage of Alzheimer disease (FAST level 7C) and does not communicate in any fashion. When asked, "Are you short of breath?" he replies with incomprehensible sounds. The NP and staff nurse observe the following behaviors: respiratory rate at 28 breaths/min, heart rate at 120 beats/min, a slight rise in the clavicles on inspiration, and a slight grunting sound at end-expiration. Additionally, he is agitated, pulling at his wrist identification band and sticking his feet out between the side rails. The nurses conclude that Wilbur is probably dyspneic, might have unrelieved pain, and is delirious.

Frances has advanced COPD (FEV$_1$ 35%) and has declined further use of mechanical ventilation. On rounds she is able to point to a vertical dyspnea visual analog scale and indicate that her dyspnea is at 30 on a 0 to 100 scale; she reports a score of 50 when she is active such as when walking to the bathroom. She is tachypneic at 28 breaths/min but a review of her vital sign flow sheet shows this as her baseline respiratory rate. The nurses conclude that Frances has mild dyspnea.

Celeste is comatose. She displays no signs of pain or dyspnea, which is no grimacing, muscle tension, clenched fists, tachycardia, tachypnea, accessory muscle use, paradoxical breathing, nasal flaring, or a fearful facial display. A soft gurgling sound is heard during respiration signifying the probability of retained upper airway secretions. Celeste has no distress.

Thomas *is vomiting when the team makes rounds. He has vomited 4 times in 8 hours and there is a fecal odor to the emesis. He is tachycardic, diaphoretic, pale, and holding his abdomen while grimacing. He reports abdominal pain at a numeric scale level of 8/10. He further reports that the pain is continuous and worsens when he vomits or tries to get up. Thomas has severe pain and unrelieved vomiting, probably secondary to a complete bowel obstruction with fecal regurgitation.*

Susan *has unresectable abdominal/pelvic carcinomatosis secondary to ovarian cancer. She reports abdominal pain at 5 on a 10-point numeric scale, and she also reports a burning and tingling pain radiating down her left leg. Susan is already on an opioid and bowel regimen but has not had a bowel movement in 48 hours. Susan has somatic and neuropathic pain probably secondary to tumor compressing nerves to her leg and constipation.*

Clarence *is unresponsive when the nurses make rounds. He is noted to be tachypneic and tachycardic but has no facial grimacing, fearful facial expression, muscle tension, accessory muscle use, or other signs of pain or dyspnea. Clarence is in no distress.*

Elaine *is agitated and trying to climb over the side rails. Attempts to orient her are unsuccessful. She points to the wall and screams, "Get it away from me, get it away" but is unable to report what she is seeing. She has firm, distended ascites and moans when her abdomen is lightly palpated. Her respiratory rate is rapid and shallow with accessory muscle use evident. Elaine is showing signs of agitated delirium with hallucinations, mild dyspnea probably secondary to loss of vital capacity from abdominal distention, and abdominal pain.*

John *has NYHA stage IV heart failure (EF 10%). He reports dyspnea only on exertion and no pain. He reports that his last bowel movement was 3 days ago. He has no appetite and wants only water to drink. John is constipated and anorexic with dyspnea on exertion.*

WHAT CAN BE DONE TO RELIEVE SYMPTOMS WITH MEDICATIONS AND BESIDES MEDICATION?

In the hospital a number of unpleasant and painful procedures and treatments are part of routine care. Limiting, eliminating, or modifying these interventions will reduce the patient's iatrogenic discomfort. A benefit-burden assessment of interventions is appropriate when the patient is terminally ill or dying and the treatment goals are to focus on patient comfort (Table 4-3).

Table 4-3 Common Hospital Interventions and Use in Terminally Ill Patients

Intervention	Action	Rationale
Arterial blood gas measurements	Discontinue, use noninvasive methods if needed, such as peripheral oxygen saturation via pulse oximetry.	Noninvasive methods are reliable estimates and are not painful.
Arterial pressure monitoring	Discontinue	No aggressive treatment of hypotension is planned.
Central venous cannulation	Discontinue if there is another peripheral venous access.	Central lines are uncomfortable compared to peripheral access.
Dressing changes	Change to an "as needed" (prn) interval. Premedicate with an analgesic before painful dressing changes.	The goal is to keep the patient dry and minimize odors. Thus, prn changes are sufficient.
EKG monitoring	Discontinue	There is no need to monitor cardiac activity when resuscitative measures are being withheld.

(Continued)

Table 4–3 Common Hospital Interventions and Use in
Terminally Ill Patients (*Continued*)

Intervention	Action	Rationale
Intracranial pressure monitoring	Discontinue	There is no need to monitor cranial pressures when brain resuscitation attempts have ceased.
Sequential compression devices	Discontinue	These can be unpleasant especially if the patient has leg pain, peripheral neuropathy, or peripheral edema.
Suctioning	Minimize frequency	Suctioning should only be done if the patient has a large volume of pulmonary or pharyngeal secretions and cannot clear the airway.
Turning	Minimize frequency, optimize positioning	Patient may have one position that optimizes pain or respiratory comfort. Frequent turning to prevent pressure ulcers may be more painful than beneficial.
Venipunctures	Discontinue	There are no lab tests that indicate distress or comfort. Metabolic derangements are expected and inevitable.
Vital sign measurements	Minimize frequency	Continued measurement helps with distress assessment and categorizing patient stability for discharge. At least once every 8 hours is useful.
Wound debridement	Discontinue	Pain exceeds benefit.

Symptom management is an art as well as a science. Finding the correct medication at the optimal dose and frequency may require frequent adjustments and frequent nursing assessments. When the patient is unaccustomed (naïve) to analgesic medications, especially opioids the standard approach is to "start low and titrate slowly" until the patient reports or displays comfort.

Pain Management[12]

Mild pain may respond well to acetaminophen and it is the first choice for treating pain in the elderly. For bone or muscle pain a nonsteroidal anti-inflammatory drug (NSAID) such as ibuprofen is often helpful. Neuropathic pain (burning, tingling, electrical) is often treated with anticonvulsants (e.g., gabapentin) in combination with other analgesics.

Moderate or severe pain often requires the use of an opioid analgesic. Short-acting agents, such as morphine, hydromorphone, or fentanyl are prescribed on either a prn basis or around the clock. Doses and dosing intervals are chosen based on the patient's pain type and needs. For example, when pain is continuous around-the-clock dosing is recommended.

When the patient reports pain relief the previous 24-hour dose of short-acting medication is converted to an equianalgesic long-acting agent, such as morphine sustained release (SR) or a fentanyl transdermal patch. A clinical pharmacist or pain specialist may be consulted to assist the prescribing clinician with making conversions. Additionally, short-acting intravenous or parenteral opioids can be converted to oral agents if the patient can swallow. Since different formulations may have differing effects on the patient it is customary to reduce the equianalgesic estimated dose of the new agent by 25%. Similarly, prn doses for breakthrough pain are usually prescribed at 10%–20% of the 24-hour opioid dose. (See Appendices N and O for opioid dosing recommendations and equianalgesia conversion information.)

Clinical Alert
Parenteral and oral morphine doses are not equivalent. There is a 1:3 parenteral-to-oral ratio. Thus 10 mg of intravenous morphine is equivalent to 30 mg of oral morphine.

Opioid-induced constipation can be avoided by beginning a bowel regimen whenever opioids are prescribed, such as a softener and/or laxative taken once or twice daily. Additionally, the patient should drink plenty of fluids, if able.

Other interventions that may reduce a patient's pain are to control the environment by decreasing lights, noise, unpleasant odors, and traffic. Complementary or alternative methods may be helpful in combination with medication. Examples include:

- Heat or cold
- Massage
- Therapeutic touch
- Acupressure
- Acupuncture
- Relaxation
- Visualization, guided imagery
- Distraction
- Music therapy

Clinical Alert
Consultation with a pain specialist or palliative care consultant is indicated when the patient has refractory pain.

Wilbur *might have unrelieved pain. His Foley catheter and wrist band are removed because he is pulling at them and they may be making him uncomfortable. The staff nurses are advised to minimize vital sign frequency, turning, and decubitus ulcer dressing changes. Acetaminophen elixir, 650 mg every 12 hours, is ordered along with morphine elixir 15 mg before dressing changes.*

Thomas *is reporting severe pain (8/10). He cannot swallow secondary to bowel obstruction and fecal vomiting so an intravenous route is chosen. Thomas had been previously comfortable with morphine SR at 60 mg every 8 hours around the clock which is 180 mg/24 hours. The equianalgesic parenteral dose is $^1/_3$ of the oral dose so Thomas needs 60 mg intravenously/24 hours (180 mg/3 = 60 mg) or 2.5 mg/hr. Adjusting by 25% for safety, the NP prescribes 45 mg intravenously/24 hours as a continuous infusion at an hourly dose of 2mg/hr. Thomas is given an intravenous bolus of 5 mg before the infusion is started. The order authorizes the staff nurse to titrate the infusion to the patient's report of pain by giving a breakthrough dose (50%–100% of the hourly rate) and increasing the infusion by this amount, every 15 minutes prn until the patient reports relief.*

Susan *has somatic and neuropathic pain. She is currently receiving morphine SR at 45 mg every 8 hours. In the past 24 hours she has used a cumulative total of 30 mg of morphine immediate release (IR) for breakthrough pain. Thus, her total need in the last 24 hours was 165 mg ([45 mg x 3]+ 30 mg) and divided by 3 for every 8-hour dosing she needs her medication changed to morphine SR at 50 mg; she will continue to get morphine IR prn for breakthrough pain. In addition, gabapentin is started in addition to morphine to attempt to relieve her neuropathic pain.*

Elaine *has distended, firm ascites and abdominal pain. She also has hepatorenal failure thus is likely to have significant delayed clearance of medication. She has no history of opioid use. Therefore, the NP prescribes morphine 4 mg intravenous push every 2 hours prn signs of pain. Around-the-clock dosing in this patient could lead to morphine toxicity.*

Dyspnea Management

Dyspnea is treated by optimizing the management of the underlying condition. For example, continuing the patient's inotropes and diuretics will prevent dyspnea when the patient has heart failure. Bronchodilators are the mainstay of current drug therapy for COPD. They are given on an as-needed basis or on a regular basis to prevent or reduce symptoms. The principle bronchodilator treatments are short- and long-acting β_2-agonists (albuterol, salmeterol), anticholinergics (ipratropium), and theophylline usually used in combination. While theophylline is effective in treating COPD inhaled bronchodilators are preferred because of the potential toxicity from theophylline.[13] Additionally, long-term oxygen therapy (>15 hours/daily) reduced mortality and improved the quality of life in patients with severe COPD who had chronic hypoxemia (PaO_2 <55 mm Hg).[14] Other strategies are directed at relieving the sensation of dyspnea and the associated emotional response and these may be effective singly or in combination (Table 4-4).

The doses of opioids for dyspnea are less well-known than those used to treat pain. As with pain management, opioids should be started at low doses of an IR form given intravenously or orally and repeated every 15 minutes until the patient reports relief. Around-the-clock dosing may be best if the patient is dyspneic continuously or at rest, with prn dosing for the patient who has episodic dyspnea.

Wilbur might be dyspneic so the nurses raise him to a 45-degree upright position and place nasal oxygen at 2 l/min. Wilbur pulls the oxygen off which suggests that he finds the cannula uncomfortable. Forcing him to wear the oxygen will cause Wilbur to expend more energy and consume more oxygen by fighting than if the oxygen is left off. He receives 3 mg of intravenous morphine and after 15 minutes is less agitated and his heart and respiratory rates are at baseline. There are already plans to give

Table 4-4 Dyspnea Interventions, Mode of Action, and Rationale

Intervention	Mode of Action	Rationale
Optimal positioning, usually upright with arms elevated and supported	Increased pulmonary volume capacity	Increases air exchange which may improve oxygenation and carbon dioxide clearance
Balance rest with activity	Decreases excessive oxygen consumption	Prevents hypoxemia
Oxygen by nasal cannula not to exceed 4 l/min	Improves oxygen saturation and delivery	Face masks may make the patient feel suffocated and cannulae are better tolerated. Nasal oxygen burns and dries nasal membranes if the flow is too high or the flow is not humidified. Some patients may not need oxygen if near death and no signs of respiratory distress.
Opioids (e.g., morphine or fentanyl)	Uncertain, may have a direct effect on *mu* receptors in the lungs.	Low doses titrated to the patient's report of dyspnea or display of dyspnea behaviors is effective.[15]
Benzodiazepines (e.g., lorazepam or midazolam)	Anxiolysis	Fear or anxiety may accompany dyspnea. Benzodiazepines have been found effective.[16]

him 15 mg of morphine elixir prn dressing changes, so the morphine order is modified to morphine elixir 15 mg by mouth before dressing changes and every 2 hours prn signs of pain or dyspnea.

Frances has mild, episodic dyspnea. She has reported worsening distress when active. Thus, her nursing care is staggered, especially on day shift, to allow rest between activities. Frances uses nasal oxygen continuously at home at 2 l/min and this is continued in the hospital along with her bronchodilators. Morphine IR 10 mg every 2 hours prn dyspnea is prescribed.

Elaine has mild dyspnea probably secondary to a loss of lung volume secondary to her ascites. Thus, upright positioning with her arms elevated may be useful. She is going to receive morphine 4 mg IV every 2 hours prn for pain and this may be a useful dose to treat dyspnea as well.

John reports dyspnea only on exertion. His inotropes and diuretics are continued to prevent pulmonary edema and dyspnea. Additionally, he is counseled about balancing rest with activity. Lastly, morphine IR 10 mg every 2 hours prn dyspnea is ordered.

Nausea/Vomiting/Diarrhea Management

Nausea can be difficult to control. The treatment is often directed at the cause and different medications may be useful (Table 4-5).

Other measures that will relieve patient distress from nausea and vomiting are:

- Frequent oral care especially after each emesis
- Cool, damp cloths to forehead
- Minimize noxious odors or sights in patient room (e.g., remove emesis promptly)

Table 4-5 Causes of and Medications for Nausea

Causes	Preferred Medication
Small bowel obstruction	Anticholinergics (e.g., scopolamine)
Gastric stasis or ileus	Prokinetic agents (e.g., metoclopramide)
Opioid-induced	Butyrophenones (e.g., haloperidol)
Complete bowel obstruction	Octreotide acetate

Vomiting that occurs from complete bowel obstruction may require nasogastric (NG) decompression or a percutaneous endoscopic gastrostomy (PEG) tube for drainage. Diarrhea may be a sign of fecal impaction and rectal examination should precede prescription of an antidiarrheal agent. A topical skin barrier may be useful if the patient is incontinent of frequent loose stools to prevent skin excoriation.

Thomas has nausea and fecal vomiting secondary to a complete bowel obstruction. An NG tube is placed and surgery is consulted about the possibility of PEG placement. Thomas's nausea is reduced by emptying his stomach, removing evidence and odors from emesis from his room, laying him flat in bed with a cool cloth on his forehead.

Constipation Management

Terminally ill patients are at very high risk of becoming constipated secondary to:

- Decreased mobility
- Decreased fluid intake
- Medication side effects (e.g., opioids)

Putting the patient on a bowel regimen to prevent constipation will include encouraging fluids, a stool softener, and perhaps a laxative (e.g., senna). Daily assessment of bowel movement frequency and completeness will guide subsequent treatment. Disimpaction and enemas may be necessary if the patient presents with severe constipation.

Susan has reported no bowel movement in 48 hours in spite of a bowel regimen. An additional laxative is added (lactulose). Susan likely has decreased GI motility secondary to tumor compression.

John has not had a bowel movement for 3 days. A rectal exam discloses no impaction. A one-time dose of lactulose is given and a daily bowel regimen of senna is started.

Table 4–6 Interventions to Reduce Anorexia and Rationale

Interventions	Rationale
Identify patient likes and dislikes	Providing pleasant, desirable, favorite foods may prompt eating
Small, frequent meals on small plates	Early satiety is common
Offer nourishment but do not force	Patients who eat to please caregivers often experience worsening nausea and vomiting.[17]
Progestational agents (e.g., megestrol)	Improves appetite and sense of well-being
Prokinetic agents (e.g., metoclopramide)	Increases gastric motility

Anorexia Treatment

Anorexia is common in patients who are approaching the end of life. During the active dying stage there is no treatment required; moreover, encouraging oral intake or providing enteral nourishment may be more burdensome than beneficial since the patient has decreasing GI perfusion. Anorexia is often the signal to clinicians that the patient has entered the active dying phase of their terminal illness.

Anorexia can also be a problem for patients who are not actively dying. Common causes include medication effects (e.g., chemotherapy), unrelieved pain, and decreased mobility, along with decreased GI motility. Interventions are various (Table 4-6).

John reports anorexia which is probably secondary to decreased GI perfusion secondary to hypotension and decreased mobility. John is offered small, frequent meals according to his personal likes and dislikes. When he doesn't eat he is not forced and his tray is removed promptly.

Delirium Management

Delirium that is not agitated and does not induce fear in the patient does not require treatment. Reducing environmental stimuli may help to reduce delirium, especially at night.

Agitated delirium puts the patient at risk of falls or self-harm. Restraints will worsen the agitation and should be employed only as a last resort. Neuroleptic medications (e.g., haloperidol), are highly effective at reducing agitated delirium in the terminally ill patient. Benzodiazepines can also be effective but their action is sedation, thus, a neuroleptic that modifies behavior may be the best first choice so the patient and family can continue interaction. (See Appendix P.)

Wilbur has agitated delirium. The NP prescribes haloperidol 2.5 mg orally every 6 hours. Wilbur is moved to a room closer to the nursing station for closer observation. His room lights are turned off, and a sign is placed on his door reminding hallway traffic to reduce noise.

Elaine has agitated delirium with hallucinations. Haloperidol is given intravenously for immediate action with good results. As with Wilbur, interventions to reduce environmental stimuli are employed. Since, Elaine has hepatorenal failure her haloperidol is prescribed prn to avoid toxicity.

Retained Upper Airway Secretions

This is a common finding during a patient's last hours as the pharyngeal muscles relax and the patient's consciousness diminishes leading to pooling of secretions in the oropharynx. It is not known whether this causes the patient distress, but families are often concerned when they hear the "death rattle." Retained airway secretions can be managed by changing the patient's position to promote drainage, reducing or eliminating intravenous hydration, and adding topical, subcutaneous, or parenteral anticholinergic drugs such as glycopyrolate or scopolamine. Suctioning is not recommended unless there is a large volume of easily reached secretions because it such a burdensome intervention.

WILL PATIENTS BECOME ADDICTED IF THEY TAKE OPIOIDS? HOW DO WE GIVE OPIOIDS TO THE PATIENT WHO IS A SUBSTANCE ABUSER? WILL OPIOIDS HASTEN DEATH?

Terminally ill patients may become tolerant of lower doses of opioids and need their medication increased to compensate for tolerance. Increasing needs do not signify addiction and patients and families need to understand that addiction is a complex psychological/social phenomenon. Patients who are accustomed to opioids or use illicit opioids will need stronger doses to achieve analgesia when experiencing pain while terminally ill. Consultation to a pain specialist may be useful in this more complicated situation.

Opioids have been the mainstay for treatment of pain and dyspnea at the end of life. There is no evidence that these medications hasten death if principles of analgesia use are followed, including

- Frequent symptom assessment
- Start low and titrate slowly (e.g., every 15 min)
- Begin an opioid regimen with short-acting opioids then convert to sustained-release formulations
- When changing agents or changing formulations adjust the equianalgesic dose down by 25% for safety
- Provide breakthrough analgesia at 10%–20% the 24-hour dose
- Escalate doses only when there is evidence (patient report or clinical signs) that distress is increasing

WHAT CAN BE DONE WHEN THE PATIENT'S SYMPTOMS ARE REFRACTORY TO TREATMENT?

Symptoms that are refractory to treatment are rare. However, after all treatment options have been exhausted, palliative sedation may be the treatment of last resort. Palliative sedation is also known as complete or terminal sedation. With the patient's or surrogate's consent a benzodiazepine or barbiturate medication is given to induce unconsciousness so that the patient loses awareness of their troubling symptoms and the patient remains unaware until natural death occurs (see Appendix Q).

Julia Wheeler, RN is assigned to care for Willard Scotia, an 89-year-old man dying from complications of terminal-stage Alzheimer disease. Mr. Scotia's 86-year-old wife has been taken home by her grandchildren. She is hard of hearing and in frail health. Before the Scotia family went home, Julia asked about phone notification in case Mr. Scotia died overnight. A granddaughter agreed to take the call and said that she would drive to her grandmother's home to make an in-person notification. She gave Julia a home phone number and a cell phone number that Julia recorded in the patient's chart. Julia also noted the family preference to call the granddaughter first.

WHEN CAN THE PATIENT BE AN ORGAN OR TISSUE DONOR?

Organ donation occurs while a brain dead patient is still being supported with fluids, medications, and mechanical ventilation to keep the organs perfused and functional. After next of kin consent is obtained the patient is taken to the operating room (OR) while still supported and the live organs are removed. The life supports are turned off after the heart and lungs have been removed.

Some patients who are near-death and supported with mechanical ventilation can also become donors. This process is called Donation after Cardiac Death (DCD). After consent is obtained, usually from a family member, the patient is taken to the OR or somewhere nearby such as the postanesthesia unit for ventilator withdrawal. After death, if the patient dies in 90 minutes or less, the body is taken to the OR for kidney and/or liver removal; these organs can tolerate a short period of no perfusion.[18]

The Centers for Medicare and Medicaid services (CMS) has enacted guidelines for consistent processes around organ donation (see Appendix K). Hospital staff must notify their state Organ Procurement Organization (OPO) when decisions about ventilator withdrawal are being considered. The OPO will collaborate with the hospital staff to identify if the patient is a donor candidate and to seek consent from the next of kin. This evaluation by the OPO must be completed before ventilation is withdrawn. This is called an imminent death notification.

When the patient is not on mechanical ventilation they are not candidates for organ donation but might be suitable to donate corneas, eyes or other tissues such as skin, heart valves, and bone after death. CMS requires that the OPO be notified after all patient deaths so that screening can be done to identify tissue donors. This is called a routine notification. The hospital and OPO have collaborative processes in place for seeking consent for organs or tissues when the patient is medically suitable.

Mr. Scotia is not on a ventilator so he is not an organ donor candidate. At his advanced age he is not likely to be a tissue donor, but only the OPO can make that designation. When Mr. Scotia dies the OPO will need a routine notification of his death and will ask the caller questions about his age, gender, race, and diagnosis.

WHO CAN PRONOUNCE THE PATIENT'S DEATH?

State law and/or hospital policy guides death pronouncement. In some states, registered nurses or advance practice nurses can pronounce death. The following are the steps for pronouncing death if this task is part of the nurse's scope.

1. Examine the patient for
   a. No audible heart sounds
   b. No palpable pulses

   c. No audible breath sounds

   d. No signs of inspiratory efforts

   e. Pupils are dilated and nonreactive

2. Record the findings in the patient's chart with the time of death. The time of death corresponds with the time of the examination. An example note follows.

8/6/07
0032

Patient has no pulses, pupillary reflexes, heart or lung sounds. He was pronounced dead at 0025. Family was notified by phone.

J. Wheeler, RN

WHO NOTIFIES THE FAMILY ABOUT THE DEATH? CAN A NURSE DO THIS? HOW SHOULD THE FAMILY BE NOTIFIED? WHAT SHOULD BE SAID OR NOT SAID? SHOULD THE FAMILY BE NOTIFIED BY PHONE IF THEY ARE NOT PRESENT?

Hospital policy may dictate who notifies the family. However, this type of communication is consistent with a nurse's knowledge, skills, and scope of practice. It may be ideal for a nurse who knows the patient and family to make the notification rather than someone who does not, such as an on-call physician.

When patient death is expected by the family the nurse can ask and document the family's preferences about notification. For many years, nurses have perpetuated the myth that a family who hears the bad news over the phone will drive recklessly and become injured en route to the hospital. There is no evidence to support this; a family who receives a call, such as "Come to the hospital, there has been a change for the worse" might drive recklessly to arrive before the patient dies. Suggested phrasing follows:

How to Say It

"Ms. Scotia, this is Ms. Wheeler. I am the nurse caring for your grandfather tonight. I am calling with sad news. (pause) Mr. Scotia died a short time ago, I'm very sorry about your loss."

After allowing time for grief responses, the nurse should ask if the family plans to come to view the body, and if not, provide information about what happens next.

How to Say It

"Ms. Scotia, we can keep your grandfather in his bed for about 2 hours if you and the rest of the family would like to see him. There are some forms you need to sign tonight if you return, or tomorrow if you would rather wait. He won't be in his bed tomorrow; we will send him to the morgue where he can be kept cold until the funeral home picks him up. Do you know what you want to do tonight?"

Avoid jargon or euphemisms when making a death notification. The clearest terms to use are *died, death, dying, dead.* The following terms are commonly used but are not universal and should be avoided:

• Passed or passed away
• Made a transition
• Left us or is gone
• No longer with us

Because of the prevalent use of cell phones while driving the nurse may inquire if the family member is behind the wheel and suggest that the driver pull over before breaking the news about the patient death. Even with the use of hands-free technology, the driver will still be distracted by news that evokes a strong emotional response.

When a patient's death is unexpected or when the family has expressed a preference for no phone notification, the caller should make a critical notification. Often the family member will press for more information, and a truthful answer should be given. For instance, if the family member asks "Has he died?" the nurse should reply in the affirmative. There is no way to reduce the impact of an unexpected loss. A reply such as, "We'll give you more information when you get here" is an avoidance of the direct question and implies that the patient has died. The family is best prepared, even in an unexpected loss, with honest answers to direct questions.

How to Say It

"This is Toni Marshall. I'm the nurse taking care of your wife tonight. She has had a sudden change in her condition. Can you come to the hospital so we can update you?"

WHEN IS THE DEATH REPORTED TO A MEDICAL EXAMINER OR CORONER?

State or county regulations will identify when a death is reported to a coroner or medical examiner. Usually, this happens when the cause of death is unknown, or there is evidence of trauma, homicide, or suicide or when the death occurred during surgery. When the death is a coroner's case it is customary to leave the catheters in place after death. The family will need an explanation for why the tubes have been left in.

HOW SHOULD THE BODY BE PREPARED FOR FAMILY VIEWING?

Patients often die with mouths and eyes open. Gentle attempts to close the eyes with a fingertip should happen as early as possible. Delays in closing the eyes may result in them staying open because rigor mortis begins in the smallest muscles first such as the eyelids. It is more difficult to close a patient's mouth. Sometimes, a rolled towel under the chin with the body laying flat will work. Tying the mouth closed looks silly and it is better to leave the patient's mouth open. Attempts to place the dentures in the mouth after death are unnecessary; the funeral director will be able to place them. Loose dentures in the deceased's mouth can easily be lost.

When the family arrives they should find the room tidy, lights low, the bed flat with side rails down, and the patient's body aligned in the center of the bed. All visible lines, tubes, and catheters have been removed unless the patient is a coroner's case. A clean gown and fresh linen completes the presentation (see Figure 4-4). Naturally, any secretions, drainage, urine, or stool will have been removed. Families usually want to

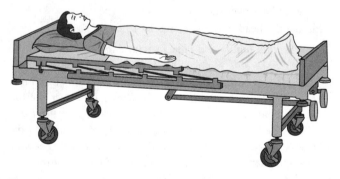

Figure 4-4   Conceptualization of a recently deceased patient prepared for family viewing.

touch, kiss, and sometimes hug the deceased so there should be no surprises under the linen.

Some families will have rituals or customs they will want to fulfill at the time of death. For example, some families will want to wash, anoint, and wrap the body with or without the nurse's assistance. Other examples of rituals include turning the bed (body) to face Mecca (the family will know the direction), saying prayers, singing, sitting with the body, clipping a lock of hair, and others. The nurse respects the importance of these traditions and finds a way to accommodate them. For example, a native American tradition involves fire and since that is not possible in a hospital room a creative nurse allowed a small votive candle at the bedside which satisfied the symbolism but maintained hospital safety codes. In some traditions the body must be buried within 24 hours of death and thus moved rapidly to a funeral home rather than being sent to the morgue.[19]

Special eye preparations must be performed before sending the body to the morgue if the patient will be donating eyes or corneas. Confirm the process with the eye bank in your community.

- Instill a few drops of normal saline in both eyes
- Tape eyes shut with paper tape avoiding the eyebrows and lashes
- Place ice bags over the eyes
- Elevate the head of the stretcher to 15 degrees

Mr. Scotia's family did plan to return to the hospital. Julie and the nurse's aide removed his Foley catheter and his nasal oxygen. He was bathed, placed in a clean gown with clean linen and positioned on his back with his arms folded over the top sheet. Equipment was removed from the room and the trash emptied. The lights were lowered as were the side rails and the door was closed in anticipation of the family's arrival. The aide placed a pitcher of water, cups, and a box of tissues on the bedside table.

Julia watched for the family and escorted them to Mr. Scotia's room. She asked if they wanted her to go in with them. Julia also offered to have the chaplain come up if the family wanted his support. When the family first entered the room, Mrs. Scotia's knees weakened and her family held her while Julia slipped a chair behind her. After a few moments Mrs. Scotia was ready to stand and approach the body. Julia stood by in case of further weakness, but remained silent to afford the family as much privacy as possible. Mrs. Scotia hugged her husband and began to cry. She sat by the bed and held his hand. She declined the chaplain. Julia left them and closed the door but peeked in often to see if anything was needed.

HOW LONG CAN THE BODY AND FAMILY REMAIN IN THE ROOM?

As a general rule, 2 hours is the average. When a cadaver remains at room temperature, bacteria begin to populate it which can produce unpleasant odors before burial; cooling the body delays this physical change. Naturally, individual patient and family circumstances will guide the amount of time, such as, distance from the hospital, weather, timeliness of notification, and others.

Families should be told as early as possible after notification about how much time the body can remain in the room. In some hospitals, special areas are available in or near the morgue for family viewing if the patient's body cannot remain in the room.

When the family is ready to leave they may need assistance gathering the patient's personal belongings. Likewise, they may have difficulty leaving. It is a poignant time to walk away and the nurse can show caring by escorting the family from the unit to the elevator or even to the door of the hospital. Other unit staff may want to extend their condolences before the family leaves. Familiarity with the family may permit a handshake or hug which is an opportunity for the family and the nursing staff to reach closure.

CLOSING VIGNETTES

Thomas gets relief from the nausea and fecal vomiting with NG decompression of his stomach. Surgery believes the risk of PEG placement is high because of carcinomatosis, shifting of the stomach from its normal position, and the patient's frail condition and hemodynamic instability. Six hours after the morphine infusion is started at 2 mg/hr Thomas reports worsening abdominal pain (10/10). The nurse gives him a bolus of 2 mg and increases his infusion to 4 mg/hr. She returns to reassess him after 15 minutes and he reports no relief. The nurse gives another bolus of 2 mg and increases the infusion to 6 mg/hr. After 20 minutes Thomas reports relief and remains comfortable through the night. He rouses easily when the nurses assess him and they recognize that oversedation would be a sign of excessive medication. The nurses assess him frequently recognizing that he may be perforating his bowel secondary to tumor invasion and his analgesia requirements are likely to escalate.

Mr. Scotia was not a candidate for tissue donation. Julia asked the family to sign a release form to authorize the funeral home of their choice to pick up the body. The family declined assistance with notifying the funeral home. Personal items from the room were gathered into a bag to take home, including the patient's dentures. Julia reminded the family that the funeral director would want the teeth when they took Mr. Scotia's clothes.

When the family was ready to leave, Julia offered a wheelchair for Mrs. Scotia, which she accepted. Julia escorted the family to the hospital door and waited with Mrs. Scotia while her grandson got the car. Hugs were exchanged and the family left.

Bobby Cartwright was struck by a car while crossing the street. He was 18 years old with no medical problems. He sustained multiple rib fractures, fractured right and left femurs, and a closed head injury. In spite of aggressive trauma care brain death was declared 24 hours after hospital admission. The designated donation requester from the OPO met with Bobby's parents

after the neurosurgeon broke the news about brain death. Bobby's
parents consented to organ and tissue donation.

For the next 24 hours the donation coordinators from the OPO
in collaboration with the intensive care unit (ICU) staff coordi-
nated Bobby's care to maintain organ integrity. Simultaneously,
the ICU nurses provided emotional support to the grieving fami-
ly and permitted unrestricted visiting. Meanwhile, lab tests were
done to match organs to recipients and transplant teams were
assembling in the OR.

The ICU nurse shooed everyone out of Bobby's room just prior
to taking him to the OR. The family gathered around the bed, and
Bobby's mother sang her son's favorite childhood song to him.
Everyone hugged and kissed Bobby and then left his room. The
family went home with assurances from the OPO coordinator
that they would be called when the surgery was finished. Bobby
was taken to the OR after his family was escorted to the door.

CLOSING PEARLS

Nurse assessment and implementation of all relevant interventions, medications and others, is key to assuring patient comfort. Patients will be unable to attend to psychological, emotional, or social needs when they have unrelieved distress.

The time of death and the immediate interval after are critical
times for the nurse to convey compassion and caring. Caring for
the body of the deceased is more than a mechanical task; the body
is a physical symbol of the deceased and as such must be cared for
in a respectful manner. Families are fragile at this time and the
nurse can have a strong positive influence on their experience.

REFERENCES

1. Solano JP, Gomes B, Higginson IJ. A comparison of symptom
prevalence in far advanced cancer, AIDS, heart disease, chronic
obstructive pulmonary disease and renal disease. *J Pain Symptom
Manage.* Jan 2006;31(1):58–69.

2. IASP Subcommittee on Taxonomy. Pain terms: a list with definitions and notes on usage. *Pain*. 1980;8:249–252.

3. Wong DL, Hockenberry-Eaton M, Wilson D, Winkelstein ML, P. S. *Wong's Essentials of Pediatric Nursing*. 6th ed. St. Louis: Mosby; 2001.

4. Puntillo KA, Morris AB, Thompson CL, Stanik-Hutt J, White CA, Wild LR. Pain behaviors observed during six common procedures: results from Thunder Project II. *Crit Care Med*. 2004;32:421–427.

5. American Thoracic Society. Dyspnea. Mechanisms, assessment, and management: a consensus statement. American Thoracic Society. *Am J Respir Crit Care Med*. Jan 1999;159(1):321–340.

6. Gift A. Validation of a vertical visual analogue scale as a measure of clinical dyspnea. *Rehabil Nurs*. 1989;14:323–325.

7. Campbell ML. Terminal dyspnea and respiratory distress. *Crit Care Clin*. Jul 2004;20(3):403–417.

8. Campbell ML. Fear and pulmonary stress behaviors to an asphyxial threat across cognitive states. *Res Nurs Health*. Dec 2007;30(6):572–583.

9. Campbell ML. Respiratory distress: A model of responses and behaviors to an asphyxial threat for patients who are unable to self-report. *Heart & Lung*. in press.

10. Beaupre' MG, Cheung N, Hess H, eds. *La reconnaisance des expressions emotionelles faciales par des decodeurs africains, asiatiques et caucasiens*; 2000. 2nd annual conference of La Societee Quebecoise de recherche en psychologie.

11. Kress JP, Hall JB. Delirium and sedation. *Crit Care Cli*. 2004;20(4):419–434.

12. Paice JA. Pharmacologic management of pain. In: Panke JT, Coyne P, eds. *Conversations in Palliative Care*. 2nd ed. Pittsburgh, PA: Hospice and Palliative Nurses Association; 2006:91–100.

13. GOLD Expert Panel. Global initiative for chronic obstructive lung disease. www.goldcopd.org

14. Tarpy SP, Celli BR. Long-term oxygen therapy. *N Engl J Med*. 1995;333:710–714.

15. Jennings AL, Davies AN, Higgins JP, Gibbs JS, Broadley KE. A systematic review of the use of opioids in the management of dyspnea. *Thorax*. Nov 2002;57(11):939–944.

16. Sironi O, Sbanotto A, Banfi MG, Beltrami C. Midazolam as adjunct therapy to morphine to relieve dyspnea? *J Pain Symptom Manage.* Mar 2007;33(3):234–236.
17. McCann RM, Hall WJ, Groth-Juncker A. Comfort care for terminally ill patients: the appropriate use of nutrition and hydration. *JAMA.* 1994;272:1263–1266.
18. Kelso CM, Lyckholm LJ, Coyne PJ, Smith TJ. Palliative care consultation in the process of organ donation after cardiac death. *J Palliat Med.* Feb 2007;10(1):118–126.
19. O'Gorman SM. Death and dying in contemporary society: an evaluation of current attitudes and the rituals associated with death and dying and their relevance to recent understanding of health and healing. *J Adv Nur.* 1998;27:1127–1135.

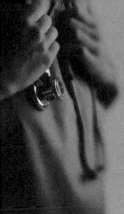

WITHDRAWAL OF LIFE-SUSTAINING DEVICES AND INTERVENTIONS

Stanley Williamson collapsed at home and was taken by ambulance to the hospital. He was unstable and unable to protect his airway so he was intubated and placed on mechanical ventilation in the emergency department (ED) before admission to the intensive care unit (ICU). He was found to have a left middle cerebral artery ischemic stroke that initially left him unresponsive with a right hemiplegia. The neurologist informed Mrs. Williamson that her husband had an 80% chance of dying from this stroke and if he survived only a 40% chance of functional recovery. The neurologist explained further that it was too soon to predict the outcome but in 3 or 4 days she would be able to make a more reliable prognosis.

Three days after ICU admission, Mr. Williamson remained comatose and the CT scan of his brain revealed cerebral edema with mass effect and impending herniation. Mrs. Williamson and their children agreed with the neurologist's recommendation to change treatment goals to a focus on comfort and to withdraw mechanical ventilation and other life supports.

We will follow this ventilator withdrawal case throughout this chapter.

❓ Frequently Asked Questions

- What is withdrawal of life-sustaining devices and interventions?

- Are we killing the patient when we stop life supports?
- What preparations need to be made before ceasing life-sustaining devices?
- What is the process for ventilator withdrawal?
- What is the process for stopping vasoactive medications, pacemakers, implantable defibrillators, or ventricular assist devices?
- What is the treatment plan for the patient who ceases dialysis?
- Do patients starve when artificial nutrition is stopped?
- Does dehydration cause distress when artificial hydration is stopped?

WHAT IS WITHDRAWAL OF LIFE-SUSTAINING DEVICES AND INTERVENTIONS?

Withdrawal of life-sustaining devices and interventions occur in spite of deteriorating vital signs, and the patient's death is expected to follow. Reasons for withdrawal include:

- Patient makes an informed, capable decision to stop prolongative measures because
  — death is imminent, or
  — quality of life is poor, or
  — devices and interventions are more burdensome than beneficial.
- Patient's surrogate makes an informed, patient-centered decision to stop prolongative measures because
  — death is imminent, or
  — quality of patient's life is believed to be poor, or
  — surrogate knows patient would not want prolongative treatment.

Ventilator Withdrawal Case—Comatose Patient

Mechanical ventilation and other life supports are being withdrawn from Mr. Williamson because death is imminent from cerebral edema and intracranial hypertension, in spite of prolongative measures.

> ### Box 5-1 Legal and Ethical Consensus about Withdrawal of Life-Sustaining Devices and Interventions
>
> - Health-care professionals serve patients best by maintaining a presumption in favor of sustaining life, while recognizing that capable patients are entitled to forgo any treatments, including those that sustain life.
>
> - Whether a treatment is warranted depends on its usefulness or benefits for a particular patient through consideration of the burdens that the treatment would impose.
>
> - An appropriate surrogate, ordinarily a family member, should be named to make decisions for patients who have insufficient capacity to make their own.
>
> - Capable patients have a common-law and constitutional right to refuse treatment.
>
> - Incapable patients have the same rights as capable patients; however, the manner in which these rights are exercised is, of necessity, different.
>
> - The decision-making process should generally occur in the clinical setting without recourse to the courts.
>
> - Artificial nutrition and hydration is a medical treatment and may be withheld or withdrawn under the same conditions as any other form of medical treatment.

Adapted from Ref. 8.

Mrs. Williamson was able to report to the neurologist that her husband had made previous statements about wanting to die naturally rather than tethered to machines.

ARE WE KILLING THE PATIENT WHEN WE STOP LIFE SUPPORTS?

There is a long-standing legal and ethical consensus that distinguishes the withdrawal of life-sustaining devices and interventions from *killing*. *Killing* is morally and legally prohibited, while *letting die* is acceptable. Killing refers to actions which are the direct causation of another's death, such as shooting with a gun or injecting potassium chloride intravenously, while allowing dying is the intentional avoidance of interventions in situations in which disease or injury causes a natural death. Allowing a natural death means to *withhold* or *withdraw* life-sustaining devices and interventions, also known as life supports[1] (Box 5-1).

WHAT PREPARATIONS NEED TO BE MADE BEFORE CEASING LIFE-SUSTAINING DEVICES?

The Centers for Medicare and Medicaid Services (CMS) has enacted guidelines for consistent processes around organ donation. Hospital staff must notify their state Organ Procurement Organization (OPO) when decisions about ventilator withdrawal are being considered (see Appendix K). The OPO will collaborate with the hospital staff to identify if the patient is a donor candidate and to seek consent from the next of kin. This evaluation by the OPO must be completed before ventilation is withdrawn. The following content is about ventilator withdrawal if the patient is not a donor.

A number of patient and family considerations are appropriate before life supports are withdrawn[2] (Table 5-1).

Table 5-1 Prewithdrawal Patient and Family Considerations and Nursing Actions

Patient and Family Considerations	Nursing Actions
What time of day is convenient for the family and the clinical team?	• Identify which team members will be present during withdrawal • Communicate the planned time to all clinical team members • Adjust the assignment so the patient's nurse can provide 1:1 patient and family care during withdrawal • Recommend the day shift to the patient's family since more hospital support staff are present
Does the family want to be with the patient during withdrawal?	• Move the patient into a private room, if available • Place chairs, boxes of tissues, and ice water in the patient's room • Arrange a private waiting area nearby for the family member(s) who don't want to be at the bedside • Obtain phone numbers from the family if they choose to leave the hospital • Ascertain who should be called first and if news of patient's death can be broken over the phone and document family choices
Are there any religious observances or other rituals that need to occur before withdrawal?	• Arrange for a chaplain or other clinical person to facilitate observances or rituals • Provide privacy during observances with a closed door or screening curtains
What is the family expecting to occur? How should the nurse prepare the family?[2]	• Ascertain family information needs • Explain about usual patient behaviors • Emphasize that the clinicians will focus on ensuring that the patient is comfortable

Mrs. Williamson and her children opted to be at Mr. Williamson's bedside during ventilator withdrawal. She reported that they were observant Roman Catholics and the Sacrament of the Sick was an important religious observance. The nurse contacted the on-call priest who came and performed the Sacrament. Mr. Williamson was already in a private room in the Neurologic ICU, but extra chairs, tissues, and water were brought to the bedside. Explanations were given about the process and the patient's responses.

How to Say It

"Have you experienced an event like this before? What was that like?"

"Shall I explain what we will be doing and what you might see?"

"Your loved one's comfort is our first priority. We may give some medication to ease uncomfortable breathing before, during or after the withdrawal process if there are signs of breathing discomfort. Breathing discomfort has a characteristic appearance, rapid breaths with a labored appearance and sometimes a fearful facial expression. We will give your loved one medication if we see those signs."

"As we turn down the ventilator your loved one will gradually take over his or her own breathing and the pattern may look different compared to when the ventilator was pushing the breaths in." (This statement should not be used if the patient is brain dead.)

"Sometimes there is coughing and mucus if we take out the breathing tube. This only lasts a short time and the patient only feels a coughing sensation."

"When the patient is close to dying the breathing will slow and sometimes there will be pauses when there are no breaths. The breaths are often shallow and some people describe them as "guppy" breaths, or the way a fish out of water breathes. This is not uncomfortable for the patient; this is the natural process of dying."

"Sometimes skin color changes from the natural color to red, or pale, or blue. These are normal changes and do not cause distress to the patient."

Clinical Alert
The state Organ Procurement Organization must be informed about the patient before mechanical ventilation is withdrawn.

WHAT IS THE PROCESS FOR VENTILATOR WITHDRAWAL?

There is very little rigorous evidence about the best processes for ventilator withdrawal, but some recommendations follow.[3] Ventilator withdrawal is usually comprised of four processes: (1) monitoring the patient before, during and after for signs of respiratory distress; (2) medicating with opioids and/or sedatives before, during and after if there are signs of patient distress; (3) reducing ventilator settings; and (4) extubation decisions.

Measuring Distress

Dyspnea is the symptom the patient undergoing ventilator withdrawal is likeliest to experience. Asking the patient who is able to report about dyspnea is the most reliable form of assessment. The patient can be asked to indicate a number, or point to a place on a visual analog scale, or nod "yes" or "no" to the question, "Are you short of breath?" (see Chapter 4).

Most patients undergoing ventilator withdrawal are unconscious, or cognitively impaired, or are too sick to self-report about dyspnea during ventilator withdrawal. Thus, patient behaviors that signify respiratory distress should be monitored, including tachypnea, accessory muscle use, paradoxical breathing pattern, nasal flaring, grunting at end-expiration, and a fearful facial expression[4,5] (Table 5-2).

Table 5-2 Operational Definitions of Respiratory Distress Behaviors

Sign	Description
Tachypnea	An increased respiratory rate, usually understood to be >24 breaths/min
Accessory muscle use	Elevation of the clavicles on inspiration with tightening of the sternocleidomastoid muscles
Paradoxical breathing pattern, also known as diaphragmatic, or abdominal, or asynchronous breathing	An inward movement of the abdomen during inspiration that is not synchronized with the outward movement of the chest
Nasal flaring	An outward movement of the distal nares during inspiration
Grunting at end-expiration	A guttural sound heard at the end of expiration. May be audible by stethoscope or without amplification
Fearful facial expression (see Figure 4-3)	(a) the upper iris is visible, (b) the teeth are visible, (c) there are lines in the forehead, (d) the eyebrows are flat, (e) the eyebrows are raised, and (f) there are no wrinkles in the nose

Medication

The medications most commonly given before, during or after ventilator withdrawal are opioids (morphine, fentanyl) and sedatives (lorazepam, midazolam). (See Appendices N, O, and P.) Some patients who are tolerant may require higher doses than patients who are opioid or sedative naïve. Doses may be given before withdrawal if respiratory distress can be anticipated. During ventilator withdrawal medications should be given intravenously for the most rapid onset of action. Documentation should include medication, dose, and indications for administration (Table 5-3).

Table 5-3 Medication Recommendations and Rationale by Patient Condition

Patient Condition	Medication Recommendation	Clinical Rationale
Brain dead	No medication	Patient is dead and unable to experience distress.
Comatose with only brainstem activity	No premedication. Bolus with morphine or a benzodiazepine during or after withdrawal if signs of distress.	Patient is unlikely to experience distress so premedication is not indicated.
Conscious and likely to have spontaneous breathing after ventilator withdrawal	Premedicate with an opioid and/or sedative. Begin a continuous infusion at 50% of the bolus dose. Titrate infusion during and after withdrawal according to patient report or signs of respiratory distress. A bolus should precede any increase in infusion rate.	Patient is likely to experience dyspnea so premedication is indicated. Patient's experience with opioids and sedatives will determine dosing and titration schedule. Bolus is needed to rapidly achieve the increased rate of infusion.
Conscious and likely to be apneic after ventilator withdrawal (high cervical quadriplegic)	Premedication essential with a barbiturate or anesthetic to achieve complete sedation.	Patient will be unable to breathe spontaneously and will experience suffocation if sedation is not complete.

Clinical Alert

*Clinical rationale, such as signs of distress, guide initia-
tion and escalation of opioids and sedatives. The
rationale, dose administered, and patient response
should be documented.*

*Mr. Williamson is comatose with no reaction to deep painful
stimuli. His pupils are nonreactive, his corneal reflexes are absent,
and there are no gag or cough reflexes. He does initiate spontaneous breaths when tested. He is not brain dead but is comatose
with only limited brainstem reflexes (breathing). Thus, he is not
premedicated before ventilator withdrawal. The nurse will monitor him closely during the process and is prepared to medicate him
with morphine if he shows signs of distress during or after
withdrawal.*

Withdrawal Methods

The three most commonly employed methods for ventilator
withdrawal include: (1) rapid terminal weaning, (2) T-bar
(T-piece) placement without weaning, and (3) no weaning
and extubation in one single step. Rapid terminal weaning
entails incremental decreases in oxygen, PEEP, and ventilation over 10–15 minutes. T-bar or T-piece placement without weaning means the ventilator is turned off. No weaning
and extubation is the most abrupt method in which the ventilator is not weaned and the patient is extubated all at one
time (Table 5-4).

*Mr. Williamson is comatose with minimal brainstem activity. His
ventilator was turned off without weaning and he is placed on a
humidified room air T-piece.*

Table 5-4 Weaning Method Recommendations and Rationale by Patient Condition

Patient Condition	Withdrawal Method Recommendation	Clinical Rationale
Brain dead	No weaning, extubation in one step	Patient is dead and unable to experience distress. Patient will not breathe or cough or gag so the airway can be removed.
Comatose with only brainstem activity	T-bar or T-piece placement without weaning or Rapid terminal weaning	Patient is unlikely to experience distress so weaning may not be necessary. Rapid weaning is an alternative approach in this patient that affords more control of clinical circumstances than the no-weaning option.
Conscious and likely to have spontaneous breathing after ventilator withdrawal	Rapid terminal weaning	This method affords the clinician the most control because the weaning process can be stopped until the patient is remediated if there are signs of distress, and then the wean progresses.
Conscious and likely to be apneic after ventilator withdrawal (high cervical quadriplegic)	Rapid terminal weaning	This method affords the clinician the most control because the weaning process can be stopped until the patient is remediated if there are signs of distress, and then the wean progresses.

Extubation Considerations

Figure 5-1 illustrates oral endotracheal tube and T-bar placement.

The endotracheal tube is an iatrogenic source of discomfort for the patient. All attempts to extubate should be made

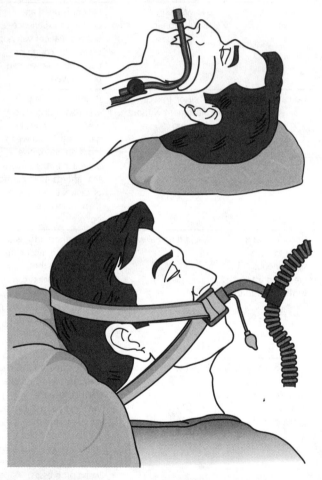

Figure 5-1   Oral endotracheal tube and T-bar setup.

Table 5-5 Extubation Recommendations and Rationale by Patient Condition

Patient Condition	Extubation Recommendation	Clinical Rationale
Brain dead	Extubate	Patient is dead and unable to experience distress. Patient will not breathe or cough or gag so the airway can be removed. Patient's physical appearance is improved without the tube.
Comatose with only brainstem activity	Extubate or retain the tube	Adequacy of cough and gag reflexes and the condition of the patient's tongue are determinative. Removal of the tube can lead to disconcerting upper airway sounds and signs of airway obstruction that may be upsetting to family and staff.
Conscious and likely to have spontaneous breathing after ventilator withdrawal	Extubate	The patient can experience distress from the tube.
Conscious and likely to be apneic after ventilator withdrawal (high cervical quadriplegic)	Extubate	The patient will not breathe so airway compromise is not anticipated.

particularly for the conscious patient. Stridor may be experienced secondary to laryngeal edema postextubation and is usually reduced by aerosolized racemic epinephrine. Some patients may need to remain intubated because of severe airway compromise that will produce signs of suffocation and be upsetting to the patient's family. When the patient's tongue is swollen and/or protuberant, or when gag and cough reflexes are absent, it may be best to retain the tube. Similarly, the tube should be retained if there is a large volume of pulmonary secretions and the patient is unlikely to experience distress from the tube (Table 5-5).

Mr. Williamson had no cough nor gag reflexes and his tongue was swollen so the oral endotracheal tube was left in place. He died 6 hours after ventilator withdrawal and never displayed any signs of distress.

Box 5-2 describes the ventilator withdrawal process for a patient who is comatose.

Box 5-2 Step-by-Step Ventilator Withdrawal Process (comatose patient)

1. Notify Organ Procurement Organization (OPO) of plans to withdraw ventilation.

2. Ascertain if family will be present and any required rituals or customs.

3. Explain the process and answer family questions.

4. Arrange for Sacrament of the Sick before withdrawing ventilation.

5. Ensure patient and family privacy with movement to a private room or shielding with curtains or screens.

6. Check IV access patency.

7. Ensure access to opioids or benzodiazepines if needed during withdrawal.

8. Have a respiratory therapist or T-piece setup on hand.

9. Turn off ventilator.

(Continued)

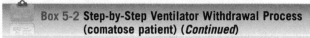

Box 5-2 Step-by-Step Ventilator Withdrawal Process (comatose patient) (*Continued*)

10. Place patient on T-piece with humidified room air.

11. Monitor for signs of respiratory distress.

12. Medicate if signs of respiratory distress.

13. Document process and patient responses.

Table 5-6 Probable Duration of Survival and Clinical Rationale by Patient Condition

Patient Condition	Probable Duration of Survival	Clinical Rationale
Multiple organ system failure	Minutes to hours	Patient has ≥3 organs in simultaneous failure and Is likely dependent on vasoactive medications as well as the ventilator.
Hemorrhage from any source	Minutes to hours	Patient will be hemodynamically unstable.
Comatose, but able to breathe spontaneously	Hours to 1 or 2 days	Respiratory drive is a powerful distal brain-stem function that persists until brain death and will support a comatose patient for many hours and sometime for more than a day.
Apneic from any cause, such as brain death, or high cervical spinal cord injury	Minutes	Patient will not breathe after the ventilator is withdrawn.

Duration of Survival

Families commonly ask the nurse about how long the patient is expected to survive after ventilator withdrawal. Duration of survival after ventilator withdrawal is difficult to predict and will depend on the number of organs in failure, blood gas exchange, and hemodynamic stability. A range of probable time can be suggested to families (Table 5-6).

How to Say It

"The usual amount of time can be predicted only in a range. For other patients with this condition we have seen survival last from ___ to ___."

"It is very difficult to predict the exact amount of time. I can tell you that usually we see a person with this condition live as short as ____ and as long as ____."

"Regardless of how long he survives his comfort and your needs will continue to be our priority."

Clinical Alert
Patient's family can be offered a predicted range about the duration of survival but must understand that the prediction is not as reliable as other clinical facts.

Ventilator Withdrawal Case—Cognitively Impaired Patient

Cecilia Rutherford was an 89-year-old nursing home resident in the advanced stage of Alzheimer disease. She slept most of the time, did not recognize or respond to her family, rarely spoke only one or two words, was incontinent of urine and stool, and was artificially nour-ished by percutaneous endoscopic gastrostomy (PEG) tube. She was rushed to the hospital after aspirating her tube feedings and was intubated in the ED and admitted to the ICU. Her family was shocked to find her on mechanical ventilation and requested with-drawal since the patient was terminally ill with a poor perceived quality of life.

Her family spent some private time with the patient and went home after giving the nurse their phone numbers. Ms. Rutherford was premedicated with morphine 5 mg intravenously and a mor-phine infusion at 2 mg/hr was initiated. The ventilator was with-drawn using a rapid weaning method, and the patient was subse-quently extubated because her cough and gag reflexes were intact. She showed no signs of distress during or after ventilator withdrawal, and the morphine infusion was continued at 2 mg/hr. Ms. Rutherford died 3 hours after the ventilator was withdrawn

Box 5-3 describes the ventilator withdrawal process for a patient who is not comatose.

Box 5-3 Step-by-Step Ventilator Withdrawal Process (cognitively impaired patient)

1. Notify OPO of plans to withdraw ventilation.

2. Ascertain if family will be present and any required rituals or customs.

3. Explain the process and answer family questions.

4. Check IV access patency.

5. Premedicate with morphine 5mg. Begin continuous infusion at 2 mg/hr.

(*Continued*)

> ### Box 5-3 Step-by-Step Ventilator Withdrawal Process (cognitively impaired patient) (*Continued*)
>
> 6. Decrease FiO$_2$ to 21% (room air).
>
> 7. Change ventilation mode to synchronized intermittent mandatory ventilation (SIMV) with pressure support ventilation (PSV) at 5 cm H$_2$O.
>
> 8. Reduce SIMV rate by 2 breaths every 3–5 minutes if no signs of distress.
>
> 9. Change ventilation mode to continuous positive airway pressure (CPAP) at 0 cm H$_2$O.
>
> 10. Turn off ventilator.
>
> 11. Extubate patient after pharyngeal and endotracheal suctioning.
>
> 12. Clean patient's face and mouth.
>
> 13. Monitor closely for signs of stridor or respiratory distress.
>
> 14. Document process and patient responses.

Ventilator Withdrawal Case—Awake Patient

Melanie White was a 62-year-old woman in the late stages of amyotrophic lateral sclerosis (ALS). Although most ALS patients forgo mechanical ventilation Mrs. White chose this intervention. After 2 years of home ventilation via a tracheostomy and PEG feedings, she was admitted to the hospital with community-acquired pneumonia and while in the hospital she made a decision for ventilator withdrawal. Her weaning parameters revealed a very low spontaneous tidal volume, as expected, and her spontaneous breathing pattern was characterized by rapid, shallow breathing, and she indicated with a finger movement that she was short of breath.

Her family (husband and children) were at her bedside and the hospital chaplain led a family prayer. Subsequently, Mrs. White was premedicated with morphine 5 mg and midazolam 4 mg, and she went to sleep. A morphine infusion at 3 mg/hr was initiated. Rapid terminal weaning was done over 15 minutes with close observation for signs of respiratory distress. At the conclusion of the weaning process, Mrs. White was placed on a tracheostomy collar with humidified room air. She did not awaken and died 20 minutes after the ventilator was turned off.

Box 5-4 describes the ventilator withdrawal process for a patient who is awake.

Box 5-4 Step-by-Step Ventilator Withdrawal Process (awake patient)

1. Notify OPO of plans to withdraw ventilation.

2. Ascertain if family will be present and any required rituals or customs.

3. Explain the process and answer patient and family questions.

4. Arrange for chaplain to lead prayer.

5. Check IV access patency.

6. Premedicate with morphine 5 mg and midazolam 4 mg. Begin continuous morphine infusion at 3 mg/hr.

7. Decrease FiO_2 to 21% (room air).

8. Change ventilation mode to synchronized intermittent mandatory ventilation (SIMV) with pressure support ventilation (PSV) at 5 cm H_2O,

9. Reduce SIMV rate by 2 breaths every 3–5 minutes if no signs of distress.

(Continued)

> **Box 5-4 Step-by-Step Ventilator Withdrawal Process (awake patient) (*Continued*)**
>
> 10. Change ventilation mode to continuous positive airway pressure (CPAP) at 0 cm H_2O.
>
> 11. Turn off ventilator.
>
> 12. Place tracheostomy collar with humidified room air.
>
> 13. Monitor closely for signs of reawakening or respiratory distress.
>
> 14. Document process and patient responses.

A ventilator withdrawal algorithm can be found in Appendix R.

WHAT IS THE PROCESS FOR STOPPING VASOACTIVE MEDICATIONS, PACEMAKERS, IMPLANTABLE DEFIBRILLATORS, OR LEFT VENTRICULAR ASSIST DEVICES?

Less is known about the best method for stopping cardiac medications and devices compared to mechanical ventilation and the following recommendations are not evidence-based given the dearth of evidence.[6] Vasoactive medications include inotropes and vasopressors (dopamine, dobutamine, norepinephrine, neosynephrine) and stopping these medications when the patient is in shock will not produce distress because the patient's blood pressure will fall causing a decrease in consciousness. Thus, these medications can be discontinued without weaning. Conversely, the conscious patient with cardiac disease may experience chest pain or pulmonary edema when dobutamine is discontinued and will require aggressive analgesia and diuresis if these symptoms develop.

Pacemakers

Cardiac pacemakers are usually implanted to treat bradycardia. The pacemaker is unlikely to prolong dying when there is multi-organ failure. Stopping a pacemaker may lead to death within minutes, especially if the patient has little or no underlying rhythm. But if the patient is not pacemaker dependent, the duration of survival is unpredictable, and the patient will need to be assessed closely for symptoms of distress. A programmer is needed to stop the functions of a cardiac pacemaker, thus a cardiology or electrophysiology consultant or a technician from the pacer company will need to be contacted to stop the pacer. Since death may follow rapidly, attention should be given to the patient and family psychological, social, and spiritual needs before pacemaker withdrawal.

Implantable Cardioverters Defibrillators

Implantable cardioverter defibrillators (ICDs) are used to prevent sudden cardiac death caused by life-threatening dysrhythmias (ventricular tachycardia, ventricular fibrillation). The ICD monitors the patient's inherent cardiac heart rate and rhythm. Based on preprogrammed settings, the ICD responds to dysrhythmias by antitachycardia pacing, cardioversion, or defibrillation. Unlike pacemakers the ICD is not operational unless the patient is experiencing a dysrhythmia, so patient distress is not produced by turning them off. However, patient distress does occur from being shocked and plans should be made to turn off the ICD when the patient is dying. As with pacemakers, a programmer is needed to stop the device.

ICD Withdrawal Case

Jacob Klein is an 82-year-old man admitted to the hospital with exacerbation of congestive heart failure (CHF). He has a history of myocardial infarctions x2, and his most recent documented ejection fraction is 15%. A year ago, he had an ICD implanted and his wife reports that it has been firing 2 to 3 times weekly in the last month. In spite of medical treatment, Mr. Klein experiences worsening renal function, decreased mentation, and cardiogenic failure.

Mrs. Klein reports her husband's previously stated wish for no prolongative treatment when he reached this illness stage. Treatment goals are changed to "comfort measures only" and Mr. Klein is transferred from the Cardiology ICU to a private room on the Palliative Care unit. Mrs. Klein and their children gather to be at his bedside. Mrs. Klein is afraid to hold his hand because she fears being shocked if his ICD fires.   Cardiology is contacted to facilitate ICD deactivation.

After deactivation the nurse reassures Mr. Klein's family that they can touch and hold him without risk of being shocked. Mrs. Klein is reminded to let the funeral director know about the device in case cremation is planned.

Ventricular Assist Devices

Ventricular assist devices (VADs) are mechanical pumps surgically implanted to improve function of the left, right, or both ventricles. Ventricular assist devices are used for patients in cardiogenic shock and for support while waiting for transplantation and sometimes as the final treatment for the rest of the patient's life. When a VAD is discontinued it is unplugged from the power source. The patient may experience heart failure with cardiogenic shock, or chest pain, or pulmonary edema. Palliative strategies to reduce distress must be in place before the VAD is turned off.

WHAT IS THE TREATMENT PLAN FOR THE PATIENT WHO CEASES HEMODIALYSIS?

When hemodialysis is stopped the patient will experience the consequences of renal failure, including uremia, hyperkalemia, and acidosis (Table 5-7). Treatment options will depend on patient consciousness, ability to experience distress, and imminence of death. For example, if the patient is comatose, a thoracentesis is more burdensome than beneficial to relieve pleural effusions.

Duration of Survival

The average survival of the hemodialysis-dependent patient is 8–10 days after the last dialysis. The patient will die sooner if he or she has cardiac or respiratory failure or septic shock. Patients who still urinate will live longer than those who are completely anuric. Patients who are in the hospital when the decision to stop dialysis is made can often be discharged to home or a nursing home with a hospice referral since death is not imminent. Individual patient circumstances along with community resources need to be considered before planning discharge. Alternatively, since the predicted duration of survival is relatively short (days) patients may be transferred to a palliative care unit or inpatient hospice bed if such exists.

Dialysis Withdrawal Case

Charles Tompkins had been on hemodialysis for 10 years before making a decision to cease treatment. He was diabetic and had experienced other complications including blindness and peripheral vascular disease. He decided to stop dialysis 3 months after undergoing an above-the-knee amputation. With his increasing physical limitations, Mr. Tompkins reported that he was ready to die.

On days 1 through 3 after the last dialysis, Charles had no serious symptoms but wanted to eat and drink "like I did before the diabetes." He was counseled to avoid too much fluid but his diet was liberalized and with enthusiasm he ate fried chicken, mashed potatoes, and fruit salad, washed down with a beer.

On day 4, he had less appetite and picked at his food. He slept more and was slow to arouse. His pruritis was relieved with skin cream and cool dressings. On day 5, a pleural rub was auscultated and Charles reported being a little short of breath. Oxygen by nasal cannula provided relief. On days 6 and 7, Charles slept continuously and was confused on awakening, and disoriented to place. His room light was kept dim and his door only slightly ajar to minimize noise. On day 8, Charles could not be roused and fine tremors were noted in his extremities. An order was placed for lorazepam prn to treat seizures.

Table 5-7 Renal Failure Pathophysiology and Patient Symptoms and Their Treatments

Pathophysiology	Patient Symptoms	Treatment
Hypervolemia Pleural effusions Pulmonary edema	Anasarca Dyspnea*	Discontinue intra-venous and enteral intake Oxygen Thoracentesis
Pericarditis Pericardial effusion	Chest pain* Malaise	Opioid analgesic prn Pericardial tap
Metabolic acidosis	Kussmaul respirations Lethargy Coma	None
Hyperkalemia	Lethargy Muscle weakness Cardiac slowing	None
Encephalopathy	Apathy Fatigue Confusion Short attention span Delirium* Seizures*	Control the environment to minimize sensory stimulation by reducing noise and lights. Neuroleptics (eg, haloperidol) Antiseizure medica-tions (eg, phenytoin or a benzodiazepine)
Gastritis	Anorexia Abdominal pain* Vomiting*	Continue antacids while awake Antiemetics
Pruritis	Itching* Excoriation*	Trim fingernails Lanolin-based lotions Cool dressings Capsaicin cream

(Continued)

Table 5-7   Renal Failure Pathophysiology and Patient Symptoms and Their Treatments (*Continued*)

Pathophysiology	Patient Symptoms	Treatment
Anemia	Fatigue Dyspnea* Chest pain*	Transfusion if death is not imminent with minimal saline flush
Peripheral neuropathy	Pain* Muscle cramps* Numbness	Gabapentin

*Symptoms that require palliation.

On day 9, the nurse noted Kussmaul respirations and bradycardia. On day 10, Charles died.

A comprehensive bibliography of references about care of the dying patient with end-stage renal disease is available at http://www.promotingexcellence.org/i4a/pages/Index.cfm?pageID=3689

DO PATIENTS STARVE WHEN ARTIFICIAL NUTRITION IS STOPPED?

When patients are unconscious or in a vegetative state they are lacking the ability to experience their internal or external environment. Thus, there is no ability to feel hungry or thirsty. The American Neurologic and Neurosurgical Association advises against beginning enteral feedings when the patient is not expected to regain a functional neurological state.[7]

For other patients, anorexia is a common experience as death approaches secondary to organ failure and the accumulation of toxic metabolites. Force feeding by tube in this patient context causes more burden than benefit. Often, it is the patient's family who experiences distress when the patient no longer wants to eat or drink. The lack of interest in food is a clear signal to the family that death is imminent and sometimes a well-intentioned family will request artificial nutrition or hydration to forestall the inevitable.

When the patient is no longer eating or drinking, or when tube feedings are stopped attention should be given to the patient's eyes, mouth, and skin as signs of dehydration may appear and be disconcerting to the family. Artificial tears, oral lubricants to the mouth, tongue and lips, and skin lotion are helpful. Furthermore, the family can be taught about applying these topical interventions and this gives the family a sense of contributing to the patient's care.

Tube Feeding Withdrawal Case

Clarence Peabody was a 28-year-old man who had been involved in a motor vehicle accident that produced a traumatic brain injury. During the initial hospitalization the prognosis for functional recovery was indeterminate so prolongative measures were initiated (tracheostomy and PEG feedings). Clarence subsequently was transferred to a long-term care facility.

After 6 months, he remained unconscious and neurologic follow up indicated that Clarence was unlikely to ever regain consciousness. His parents and siblings believed Clarence would not want to be prolonged further. Thus, his tube feedings were discontinued. Clarence continued to receive around-the-clock basic nursing care including bathing, turning, suctioning. The frequency of mouth care was increased from daily to every 8 hours and his mouth was liberally lubricated and an oral lubricant was applied to his lips. His parents visited daily and reported satisfaction with Clarence's appearance and lack of signs of distress. On day 5 after the feedings were stopped, they noted that his urine was dark and the volume was low, additionally, his eyes appeared sunken. The nurse assured the family that these were normal changes that do not cause distress. On day 9, Clarence was anuric and a Cheyne-Stokes breathing pattern was apparent. On day 10, Clarence died.

Closing Pearl

Decisions to withdraw life-sustaining devices and interventions are emotionally draining for patient and their families. The nurse is in a visible and accessible position to aid with both the physical care and the emotional support during these processes.

REFERENCES

1. Beauchamp TL, Childress JF. *Principles of biomedical ethics.* 4th ed New York: Oxford University Press; 1994.
2. Kirchhoff KT, Conradt KL, Anumandla PR. ICU nurses' preparation of families for death of patients following withdrawal of ventilator support. *Appl Nurs Res.* May 2003;16(2):85–92.
3. Campbell ML. How to withdraw mechanical ventilation: a systematic review of the literature. *AACN Adv Crit Care.* October/December 2007;18(4):397–403.
4. Campbell ML. Fear and pulmonary stress behaviors to an asphyxial threat across cognitive states. *Res Nurs Health.* Dec 2007;30(6): 572–583.
5. Campbell ML. Psychometric testing of a respiratory distress observation scale. *J Palliat Med.* 2008;11(1):44–50.
6. Wiegand DL, Kalowes PG. Withdrawal of cardiac medications and devices. *AACN Adv Crit Care.* October/December 2007;18(4): 415–425.
7. Quality Standards Subcommittee. Practice parameters: assessment and management of patients in the persistent vegetative state. *Neurology.* 1995;45:1015–1018.
8. Meisel A, Snyder L, Quill T. Seven legal barriers to end-of-life care: myths, realities, and grains of truth. *JAMA.* Nov 15 2000;284(19): 2495–2501.

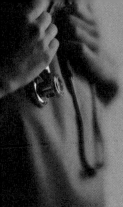

Chapter 6

ANTICIPATORY, ACUTE, AND NURSES' GRIEF

Beth Foley, RN, BSN is the charge nurse on a 15-bed medical-surgical unit. She is surprised when she enters the nursing unit at 0645 and finds family members of a dying patient standing in the hall, sitting on the hall floor, and overflowing from the patient's room. As she gets report from the night staff she learns that Mrs. Jackson's death is imminent and family has been assembling all night. As many as 25 people have been on the unit since early evening and more are expected. Mrs. Jackson is 89 years old and the matriarch of a large, extended family who lives all over the country.

We will follow this family grief case about an expected death throughout the chapter.

❓ Frequently Asked Questions

- How are anticipatory grief, acute grief, and mourning differentiated?
- What are the common manifestations of grief?
- What can I say to the family who is anticipating a death?
- How can the staff and I support the family during the patient's death?
- What rituals or customs might the grieving family want performed?

- What is complicated grief and how will I recognize families at risk?
- What makes caring for dying patients stressful for nurses?
- What are the signs of burnout?
- How can I help myself or a colleague who is stressed about caring for dying patients?

HOW ARE ANTICIPATORY GRIEF, ACUTE GRIEF, AND MOURNING DIFFERENTIATED?

- **Grief** is the emotional and physical reaction to a loss; it is a normal process expressed in individual ways.
- **Anticipatory grief** is the emotional and physical reactions to an impending loss and can be experienced by the patient and the family. It intensifies as the time of death approaches.
- **Acute grief** occurs during the loss interval (e.g., at the time of death) and is experienced by the survivors of the deceased. The intensity is expected to decrease over time.
- **Mourning** is the outward display of the internal physical and emotional feelings associated with the loss. Religious beliefs, cultural norms, and customary rituals characterize mourning behaviors.

 Clinical Alert
There is no universal grief experience. Individuals will vary even within the same family or community.

WHAT ARE THE COMMON MANIFESTATIONS OF GRIEF?

Theoretical tasks of grief have been suggested. The best known but least studied are Kubler-Ross's stages of grief: denial, anger, bargaining, depression, and acceptance that she described as defense and coping mechanisms for the patient.[1] Since Kubler-Ross other investigators have proposed theoretical tasks that occur during grieving[2] (Table 6-1).

A number of studies have described manifestations of grief that occur in one or more of the following domains: physical, cognitive, emotional, and behavioral[3] (Table 6-2).

WHAT CAN I SAY TO THE FAMILY WHO IS ANTICIPATING A DEATH?

Sometimes clinical staff avoid the family of a patient who is dying because they fear saying the wrong thing. This can lead the family to feel avoided and abandoned at a time of great need. When in doubt, saying nothing but being present may be enough.

How to Say It

"I'm feeling sad for you and your family"
"I wish I could take away your pain"
"Would you like to tell me about her?" (be sure to sit down and listen)

Phrases to avoid
"His suffering will be over soon" or "She'll be at peace soon" (trivializes family's loss)
"He's going to a better place" (belief in an afterlife is not universal)
"You can get on with your life" (trivializes both the loss and the altruism of caregiving)
"When my mother died . . ." (compels family to offer the nurse condolences)

Table 6-1 Theoretical Tasks of Grief

Kubler-Ross 1969	Parkes 1987	Bowlby 1980	Wordon 1991	Rando 1993
1. Denial	1. Alarm	1. Numbing	1. Accept reality of the loss	1. Recognize the loss and death
2. Anger	2. Searching	2. Searching and longing	2. Experience the pain of grief	2. React to, experience, and express the separation and pain
3. Bargaining	3. Mitigation	3. Disorganization and despair	3. Adjust to an environment without the deceased	3. Reminisce
4. Depression	4. Anger and guilt	4. Reorganization	4. Withdraw emotional energy and reinvest in another relationship	4. Relinquish old attachments
5. Acceptance	5. Gaining a new identity			5. Readjust and adapt to the new role while maintaining memories, and form a new identity
				6. Reinvest

Adapted from Brown-Saltzman.[2]

Table 6-2   Manifestations of Grief[3]

Physical	Cognitive	Emotional	Behavioral
Headaches	Sense of depersonalization	Anger	Impaired work performance
Dizziness	Inability to concentrate	Guilt	Crying
Exhaustion	Sense of disbelief and confusion	Anxiety	Withdrawal
Muscular aches	Idealization of the deceased	Sense of helplessness	Avoiding reminders of the deceased
Sexual impotency	Search for meaning in life and death	Sadness	Seeking or carrying reminders of the deceased
Loss of appetite	Dreams of the deceased	Shock	Overreactivity
Insomnia	Preoccupation with image of deceased	Yearning	Changed relationships
Feelings of tightness or hollowness	Fleeting visual, tactile, olfactory, auditory hallucinatory experiences	Numbness	
Breathlessness		Self-blame	
Tremors		Relief	
Oversensitivity to noise			

HOW CAN THE STAFF AND I SUPPORT THE FAMILY DURING THE PATIENT'S DEATH?

As discussed in Chapter 3, unrestricted visiting, helping with basic care, and knowing when death is imminent are important to families.

Families engaged in a vigil at the bedside often forget to eat, wash, change clothes, and get fresh air. The nursing staff can encourage families to take care of themselves by making hygiene supplies and food, water, and juices available. Encouraging the family to go home may make the family more anxious about leaving the patient and the possibility that the patient will be alone at the time of death.

Frequent checks on the family and patient are welcome even when the family has closed the door. Families are sometimes afraid to be alone with the patient or anxious that the patient may be suffering; this often leads to frequent requests for someone to check the patient. The nurse can anticipate this family need and forestall the overuse of the call bell by making frequent checks.

A well-intentioned housekeeper or maintenance person who does not know the patient-family circumstances might inadvertently say the wrong thing, such as "he's looking better today" or enter the room without knocking or during payer. The nurse needs to keep all staff on the unit aware that a death is impending and while the nurse should check on patient and family frequently, other unnecessary intrusions can be avoided. In some hospitals, a token such as a butterfly magnet, is placed on the patient's room door to alert hospital staff that a patient is dying in that room.

Family Grief Case—Expected Death

Mrs. Jackson is well known to the nursing staff after frequent hospitalizations for her many chronic medical conditions. The nurses are acquainted with the oldest daughter who cares for the patient at home and are aware that Mrs. Jackson has seven other adult children and 48 grandchildren with several great-grandchildren.

On this hospital admission, Mrs. Jackson has sustained an ischemic stroke and is not expected to survive. Her previously stated wishes to "go naturally" have led to a palliative care treatment plan with no plans to intubate or resuscitate. Mrs. Jackson was admitted to a private room and her family has been given open visiting privileges.

Beth recognizes the potential lack of privacy and confidentiality of the other unit patients with so many visitors in attendance on Mrs. Jackson. She further recognizes the need for the family to assemble and be together at this time. She makes the nursing conference room available to the family and stocks it with tissues, water, ice, and juices. The family in the hall is encouraged to move into this room and make it the family's "base." Beth explains the reason for asking the family to use this room instead of lounging in the hallway.

In addition, Beth gives the nurse assigned to Mrs. Jackson a lighter assignment because she knows that family care will consume a lot of time and patience. The entire day shift staff is alerted to keep the noise and traffic to a minimum outside Mrs. Jackson's room. See the closing vignette for additional details.

WHAT RITUALS OR CUSTOMS MIGHT THE GRIEVING FAMILY WANT PERFORMED?

Rituals and customs before and at the time of death are highly variable among and within families. Religion, ethnicity, acculturation, and setting all influence the expected customs. It would be difficult to know all the possible customs and the nurse should not make stereotypical assumptions (Table 6-3).

Table 6-3 Common Religious or Ethnic Practices during Dying or at Death

Religion or Culture	Ritual or custom	Hospital Accommodations
Catholic	Sacrament of the Sick is performed by a priest	Priest on premises or on-call
	Place rosary, medals, or scapular (a religious symbol on a string around neck) on patient	Avoid losing religious materials during bathing
Judaism[5]	Avoidance of autopsy unless required by law or organ-tissue donation unless sanctioned by a rabbi	Offer autopsy and/or donation but accept refusal
	Rapid removal of body to funeral home for burial within 24 hours of death except on the Sabbath (Saturday)	Permit funeral home staff to retrieve body from patient room
Islam[5]	Turn bed east to face Mecca	Family will know the direction
	Family members of same gender as patient prepare the body after death	Provide the requested materials, family will bring any materials that are not customarily found in the hospital
	Avoidance of autopsy unless required by law	Offer autopsy and/or donation but accept refusal
	Organ donation may be allowed	
	Rapid removal of body to funeral home for burial within 24 hours of death	Permit funeral home staff to retrieve body from patient room
Buddhism[5]	A quiet place for dying so the patient can engage in wholesome thoughts and reflection on past good efforts	Move patient to a private room

(Continued)

Table 6-3 Common Religious or Ethnic Practices During Dying or at Death (*Continued*)

Religion or Culture	Ritual or custom	Hospital Accommodations
Hinduism[5]	Family may refuse analgesics because consciousness is desirable until death	Offer doses of analgesia that will not cloud consciousness
	Turn bed so patient's head facing India (east)	Family will know the direction
	Chanting, prayer, and incense are part of the ritual	Avoid interrupting during ritual prayers
	Application of sacred ash to the patient's forehead and placing drops of sacred water from the Ganges river in the patient's mouth may be done	Do not wash ash off forehead
	Family members of same gender as patient prepare the body after death	Provide the requested materials, family will bring any materials that are not customarily found in the hospital
African American	Extended family gathers to be with patient and each other	Private room, extra chairs, a private waiting area nearby for overflow if available
	Clergy are important counselors at this time	Offer hospital chaplain support if no personal clergy visits
Latin/ Hispanic	Usually Catholic	Priest on premises or on-call
	Extended family gathers to be with patient and each other	Avoid losing religious materials during bathing
		Private room, extra chairs, a private waiting area nearby for overflow if available
Native American	Variable	Seek advice from tribal leader

Clinical Alert
Assumptions about customs and rituals should not *be made. Ask first.*

How to Say It

"Are there any rituals or customs in your family that I should know about?"
"I see your mother has a rosary. Is she Catholic? Would she want the Sacrament of the Sick?"
"I noticed your Bible. Would you like our chaplain to come and lead a prayer?"

WHAT IS COMPLICATED GRIEF AND HOW WILL I RECOGNIZE FAMILIES AT RISK?

Complicated grief does not diminish over time and can lead to withdrawal, loss of job, depression, weight loss, substance abuse, and suicidal thoughts and actions. Individuals at risk for complicated grief include family members who had an extremely intense, close relationship or were estranged from the patient, or families bereaved by suicide or homicide.

People experiencing complicated grief may need psychological therapy. Nurses who recognize the risk of complicated grief may suggest grief counseling resources to the family before the patient's death or discharge from the hospital. Most hospices provide this type of support and include any community members needing the service.

WHAT MAKES CARING FOR DYING PATIENTS STRESSFUL FOR NURSES?

Patient care is inherently stressful because nurses engage with patients during times of patient stress, and nurses often empathize with the patient and feel the stress of the patient. Some types of nursing care bring more stresses, including care of the dying. Stressors specific to care of the dying include:

- Facing the reality of own mortality[4]
- Coping with the patient's unrelieved symptoms[4]
- Witnessing family grief
- Dealing with ethical issues
- Disagreeing with the care provided by other disciplines
- Not having the skills or experience to care for the dying

In addition, all nurses are dealing with workplace stressors, including short staffing, and workplace demands.

WHAT ARE THE SIGNS OF BURNOUT?

Signs of burnout fall into four categories: physical, psychological, behavioral/social, and spiritual symptoms[4] (Table 6-4).

Table 6-4   Signs of Nurse Burnout[4]

Physical	Psychological	Behavioral/ Social	Spiritual
• Insomnia	• Anxiety	• Chemical abuse	• Doubt about beliefs
• Fatigue	• Irritability	• Avoiding patients	• Anger at God
• Decreased resistance to infection	• Increased frustration with others	• Absenteeism	• Belief that a major life change is needed, such as a new job
• Weight changes	• Feelings of alienation	• Tardiness	
• Memory problems	• Isolation	• Sarcasm	
• Muscle aches and pains	• Low self-esteem	• Derogatory labeling of patients	
• GI complaints		• Pessimism	

HOW CAN I HELP MYSELF OR A COLLEAGUE WHO IS EXPERIENCING BURNOUT?

Self-care to minimize the risk of burnout is encouraged and includes one or more of the following activities (Box 6-1).

> **Box 6-1 Lifestyle Management Techniques[6]**
>
> Recognize and monitor symptoms
> Practice good nutrition
> Use meditation
> Pay attention to your spiritual life
> Grieve losses, personally and as a team
> Decrease overtime work
> Exercise
> Spend time in nature
> Incorporate music
> Try energy work (e.g., reiki, healing touch, therapeutic touch)
> Maintain a sense of humor
> Balance work and home life to allow sufficient "time off"
> Have a good social support system, personally and professionally
> Discuss work-related stresses with others who share the same problems
> Visit counterparts in another institution; look for new solutions to problems
> Seek consultation if symptoms are severe, such as from the Employee Assistance Program if one exists at your institution or from a mental health professional

CLOSING VIGNETTES

Family Grief Case—Expected Death

Mrs. Jackson is African American with a large, extended family that all live locally. Besides her family, her pastor from her

Baptist Church has been a daily visitor. Beth asks Mrs. Jackson's caregiver daughter if there any rituals or customs that are important to the patient and her family at this time. The daughter states that singing hymns is an important tradition. Beth requests that the hymns be sung softly so as not to disturb other patients and shortly thereafter the staff are touched to hear soft, lovely family voices singing together as they circle Mrs. Jackson's bed. When Mrs. Jackson's nurse sticks her head in to check on the patient she is pulled gently into the circle and knowing the hymn she softly joins in for a chorus before excusing herself.

As the day progresses, family members move quietly back and forth from the patient's room to the conference room. Someone goes out and brings back food and the nurses keep the water, juice, and tissues replenished.

Suddenly, loud noises and crying are heard from Mrs. Jackson's room and several family members erupt into the hallway grieving expressively. While the assigned nurse enters to check the patient, Beth closes room doors of nearby patients to minimize the noise. Beth recognizes that acute grief behaviors are unique to individuals and are normal expressions of intense emotions. She knows that asking for quiet will not be successful. Instead she minimizes the disruption for other patients and gently shepherds the family into Mrs. Jackson's room or the conference room.

A physician is called to pronounce the death and the family waits in the conference room while the nursing staff cleans and lays out the body. The family sees the patient once more and leaves singly and in groups. Some are weeping quietly, others are sad but silent. Beth has explained the postdeath processes and encouraged safe driving.

Family Grief Case—Unexpected Death

Jimmie Tyler, 18 years old, was fatally injured in a car accident with other teenagers. He was unrestrained and tossed from the car. The other teens were less seriously injured and are expected to survive. Jimmie has been admitted to the Neurologic Intensive Care Unit (NICU) with a cervical spinal fracture and a traumatic brain injury. His parents, siblings, girlfriend, and other friends from school have begun to gather in the ICU waiting room. Unlike Mrs. Jackson's, Jimmie's death will be unexpected and traumatic.

Each time a new person arrives there is an upsurge of crying, screaming, and fainting in the waiting room. This is particularly disruptive to the other ICU families who do not know how to respond. The NICU is busy and short-handed and there is no one from the NICU staff who can attend to the family. Because aggressive, lifesaving measures are being performed on Jimmie, visitation is limited. This contributes to family distress, but can't be avoided.

The NICU charge nurse calls the nursing supervisor and chaplain to see if anyone can be identified to assist the family. As with Mrs. Jackson, the supervisor appropriates a nearby class-room for Jimmie's family. She recognizes their need to express grief and distress and the privacy that entails. The chaplain plans to spend as much of the day as his demands permit to sup-port the family while they await Jimmie's outcome.

Jimmie dies but his parents are at the bedside in spite of all the detritus from the failed attempt to resuscitate. His mother faints and is carried from the room where she is revived with a cool cloth to her forehead. The assembled siblings and friends from school are teenagers with teenagers' labile emotions, and they exhibit a range of expressive emotions, including crying, screaming, and anger. The chaplain stays nearby and knows that these emotions have to be let out. When the young people have exhausted themselves he offers to lead them in prayer and they agree.

The chaplain escorts the family to the hospital exit when they are ready to leave. He returns to the NICU to minister to the staff.

Although, all that could be done for this family was done, the staff does not feel the same satisfaction in a job well done as the staff caring for Mrs. Jackson. Clearly, the death characteristics influence how much a nurse can do to assuage the family's grief.

Nurse Burnout Case

Mark has worked on the neurologic unit for a year. He normally displays empathetic and caring behaviors; however, recently he has been complaining about patients' families in the report room and has been sarcastic and condescending in his descriptions. Additionally, Mark has been late returning from breaks with no apology to his colleagues.

Mark's colleagues surprised him with bagels and cream cheese during shift report the next time he worked. Over bagels they gently told him that his stress behaviors were obvious and of concern. Mark acknowledged that caring for a recent dying patient, a young person, was stressful to him because it reminded him of his deceased brother who died similarly. As a group, they agreed to avoid assigning dying patients to Mark until he reported his readiness. Similarly, the staff agreed to invite the hospital chaplain to come and provide staff support whenever there were dying patients on the unit.

Nurse Burnout Case

Marjorie is nearing retirement after 40 years giving hospital care. Five years ago she transferred from a surgical unit to the palliative care unit because of the quieter pace. Recently, she has experienced the loss of her husband and two of her siblings and she is noticeably irritable with her peers. She complains frequently that her back, legs, and feet hurt and she is slow to answer call lights preferring to stay at the desk and send someone else to respond. At the same time, she is quick to criticize the younger nurses for having no "work ethic."

For a while, the other staff has accepted Marjorie's behaviors but after a particularly busy week the manager begins to receive complaints that Marjorie is not "pulling her weight" or "doing her share."

The manager meets with Marjorie and without disclosing the peer complaints asks her how she feels about the work she is doing. Marjorie quickly identifies the need to do something else for her last year of work. She acknowledges that the complete care required by terminally ill patients is too physically demanding and the emotions are too harsh after her recent personal losses. A meeting with human resources is planned.

In this last case, it may be best for the nurse to move to a different practice area.

CLOSING PEARLS

Survivors will always remember the circumstances of a loved one's death. Nurses have the unique opportunity to influence those circumstances in a positive manner by empathetic behavior and supportive interventions.

All nurses are at risk for workplace stress. Self-care and care of colleagues should be an integral part of nursing practice.

REFERENCES

1. Kubler-Ross E. *On Death and Dying.* New York: Macmillan; 1969.
2. Brown-Saltzman K. Transforming the grief experience. In: Carroll-Johnson R, Gorman L, Bush NJ, eds. *Psychosocial Nursing Care: Along the Cancer Continuum.* 2nd ed. Pittsburgh: Oncology Nursing Press, Inc.; 2006.
3. Corless I. Bereavement. In: Ferrell BR, Coyle N, eds. *Textbook of Palliative Nursing.* 2nd ed. New York: Oxford; 2006:531–544.
4. Mazenec P. Self-care strategies. In: Panke JT, Coyne P, eds. *Conversations in Palliative Care.* 2nd ed. Pittsburgh, PA: Hospice and Palliative Nurses Association; 2004:261–269.

5. Kemp C, Bhungalia S. Culture and the end of life: A review of major world religions. *Journal of Hospice and Palliative Nursing.* 2002;4(4):235–242.
6. Vachon MLS. The experience of the nurse in end-of-life care in the 21st century. In: Ferrell BR, Coyle N, eds. *Textbook of Palliative Nursing.* 2nd ed. New York: Oxford University Press; 2006:1011–1029.

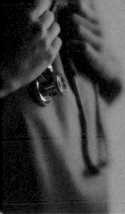

AMERICAN NURSES ASSOCIATION POSITION STATEMENT ON NURSING CARE AND DO-NOT-RESUSCITATE (DNR)* DECISIONS

SUMMARY

Nurses face ethical dilemmas concerning confusing or conflicting DNR orders and this statement includes specific recommendations for the resolution of some of these dilemmas. Although cardiopulmonary resuscitation has been used effectively since the 1960s,[1] the widespread use and possible overuse of this technique and the presumption that it should be used on all patients has been the subject of ongoing debate.[2,3] The DNR decision should be directed by what the informed patient wants or would have wanted. This demands that communication about end of life wishes occur between all involved parties [patient, health care providers (HCPs), and family; the latter as defined by the patient], and that appropriate DNR orders be written before a life-threatening crisis occurs.

BACKGROUND

Expectations that the Patient Self-Determination Act would facilitate communication about DNR orders among HCPs and patients led to a disappointing clinical reality, as research has shown low rates of advance directive (AD) completion and

---

poor ability of ADs to influence physicians' decisions about writing DNR orders.[4–6] This is partly due to the confusion surrounding how written ADs are interpreted, how DNR decisions are made and implemented, and how DNR itself is defined.[4,7,8] Some have argued that HCPs focus too narrowly on the DNR order, which typically prohibits attempts to restore cardiopulmonary function in the event of a patient's cardiac or pulmonary arrest. Instead, they assert that the focus should be on the goals of medical treatment, for example:

- Life prolongation regardless of quality;
- Comfort and symptom palliation; or
- Aggressive attempts to sustain life with the understanding that life-sustaining technology will be withdrawn if it does not meet the goals agreed upon by the HCP and patient or family.[6,9–11]

RECOMMENDATIONS

In view of the confusion and complexity that continue to surround DNR decisions and their implementation, ANA makes the following recommendations:

1. Whenever possible, the DNR decision should be a subject of explicit discussion between the patient and the family (or designated surrogate) acting according to the patient's wishes, if known, or alternately, the patient's best interest, and the health care team. The efficacy and desirability of CPR attempts, a balancing of benefits and burdens to the patient, and therapeutic goals should be considered.

2. The choices and values of the competent patient should always be given highest priority, even when these wishes conflict with those of HCPs and families. An exception to this is if CPR attempts are requested via an AD or surrogate but one or more physicians determine, as allowed by state law, that CPR attempts would not be medically effective.[12]

3. Nurses need to be aware of and have an active role in developing DNR policies within the institutions where they work. Specifically, policies should address, consider, or clarify:

- Potentially confusing orders such as "chemical code only," or "resuscitate, but do not intubate;"
- Inappropriateness of "slow codes" or "show codes" (i.e., attempts to demonstrate or mimic a response, perhaps for the benefit of family members, that stops short of a full resuscitation effort);
- Guidance to HCPs who have evidence that a patient does not want CPR attempted but for whom a DNR order has not been written;
- Required documentation to accompany the DNR order, such as a progress note in the medical record indicating how the decision was made;
- The role of various HCPs in communicating with patients and families about DNR orders;
- Effective communication of DNR orders when transferring patients within or between facilities;
- Effective communication of DNR orders among staff that protects against patient stigmatization or confidentiality breaches;
- Guidance to HCPs on specific circumstances that may require reconsideration of the DNR order (e.g., patients undergoing surgery or invasive procedures);
- The needs of special populations (e.g., pediatrics).

4. DNR orders must be clearly documented, reviewed and updated periodically to reflect changes in the patient's condition[13];

5. There should be no implied or actual withdrawal of other types of care for patients with DNR orders. Attention to language is paramount, and euphemisms such as "doing everything," "doing nothing," or "withdrawing care," to indicate the absence or presence of a DNR order should be strictly avoided;

6. Exclusive of condition-specific DNR orders[9], a patient who has a DNR order and who suffers cardiopulmonary arrest for whatever reason should not have CPR attempts performed;

7. Nurses have a duty to:
   - *educate* patients and their families about the use of biotechnologies at the end of life, termination of treatment decisions, and ADs;
   - *encourage* patients to think about end of life preferences in advance of illness or a health crisis, to discuss them with their HCP(s) and family, and to implement an AD;
   - *communicate* known information that is relevant to end of life decisions;
   - *advocate* for a patient's end of life preferences to be honored.
8. Nurses should participate in an interdisciplinary mechanism (e.g., interdisciplinary ethics committee) for the resolution of disputes among patients, families and/or HCPs concerning DNR orders.[14]

The appropriate use of DNR orders, together with adequate palliative end of life care, can prevent suffering for many dying patients who experience cardiac/pulmonary arrest. As the primary continuous HCP in health care facilities, the nurse must be involved in the planning as well as the implementation of resuscitation decisions. Clear DNR policies at the institutional level that include the basic features that ANA recommends will enable nurses to effectively participate in this crucial aspect of patient care.

*Other terms include "Do Not Attempt Resuscitation" and "no CPR"

REFERENCES

1. Kouwenhoven, W.B., Jude, J.R, & Knickerbocker, G.G. "Closed-chest cardiac massage," *JAMA*. 1960, 178:84–97
2. Hayward, M. (1996). Cardiopulmonary resuscitation: Are practitioners being realistic? *Arch Inter Medi*. 156(7):793:97
3. Lederberg, M.S. (1997). Doctors in limbo: The United States DNR debate. *Psychooncology*. 6(4):321–328
4. Hakim, R.B., Teno, J.M., Harrell, F.E., Jr., Knaus, W.A., Wenger, N., Phillips, R.S., Layde, P., Califf, R., Connors, A.F., Jr., & Lynn,

J. (1996). Factors associated with do-not-resuscitate orders: Patients' preferences, prognoses, and physician's judgments. SUPPORT Investigators. Study to Understand Prognoses and Preferences for Outcomes and Risks of Treatment. *Ann Inter Med.* 125(4):284–293.

5. Jacobson, L.J., Kasworm, E. (1999). May I take your order: A user-friendly resuscitation status and medical treatment plan form. *Qual Manage in Health Care.* 7(4):13–20.

6. Prendergast, T.J. (2001). Advance care planning: Pitfalls, progress, promise. *Crit Care Med.* 29(2 Suppl), N34–39.

7. Heffner, J.E., Barbieri, C. & Casey, K. (1999). Procedure specific do-not-resuscitate orders. Effect on communication of treatment limitations. *B J Nurs.* 8(12):810–814.

8. Teno, J.M., Stevens, M., Spernak, S. & Lynn, J. (1998) Role of written advance directives in decision making: Insights from qualitative and quantitative data. *J Gen Intern Med.* 1998 July;13(7):439–446.

9. Choudhry, N.K., Choudhry, S., & Singer, P.A. (2003). CPR for patients labeled DNR: The role of the limited aggressive therapy order. *Ann of Intern Med.* 138(1):65–68.

10. Fischer, G.S., Alpert, H.R., Stoeckle, J.D., Emanuel, L.L. (1997). Can goals of care be used to predict intervention preferences in an advance directive? *Arch Intern Med.* 157(7):801–807.

11. Kolarik, R.C., Arnold, R.M. Fischer, G.S. & Hanusa, B.H. (2002). Advance care planning. *J Gen Intern Med.* (8):618–624.

12. Ditillo, B.A. (2002). Should there be a choice for cardiopulmonary resuscitation when death is expected? Revisiting an old idea whose time is yet to come. *J Palliat Med.* 5(1):107–116.

13. Joint Commission on the Accreditation of Health Care Organizations (1992) "Nursing Care Standards," Accreditation Manual for Hospitals. Oak Bluffs Terrace, Illinois.

14. Casarett, D. & Siegler, M. (1999). Unilateral do-not-attempt-resuscitation orders and ethics consultation: A case series. *Crit Care Med.* 27(6):1116–1120.

Effective Date: 1992; Revised 1995; Revised 2003
Status: Revised Position Statement
Originated by: Task Force on the Nurse's Role in End of
                     Life Decisions
Adopted by: ANA Board of Directors
Revised by: The Advisory Board of the ANA Center for
                     Ethics and Human Rights

Related Past Action:

1. Code for Nurses With Interpretive Statements, 2001
2. Nursing and the Patient Self-Determination Act, 1991
3. Promotion of Comfort and Relief of Pain in Dying Patients, 1991

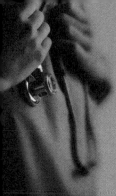

Appendix B

EXECUTIVE SUMMARY CLINICAL PRACTICE GUIDELINES FOR QUALITY PALLIATIVE CARE

FOREWORD[1-21]

Palliative care and hospice programs have grown rapidly in recent years in response to both growth in the population living with chronic, debilitating, and life-threatening illness and to clinician interest in effective approaches to the care of such patients. Palliative care is medical care provided by an interdisciplinary team, including the professions of medicine, nursing, social work, chaplaincy, counseling, nursing assistants, and other health care professions, focused on the relief of suffering and support for the best possible quality of life for patients facing serious life-threatening illness and their families. It aims to identify and address the physical, psychological, spiritual, and practical burdens of illness. This summary will present a professional consensus from five major United States palliative care organizations* on clinical guidelines for quality palliative care services. The complete document, its appendices, and a comprehensive set of references are available online at www.nationalconsensusproject.org or as a printed document, available upon request.

---

*American Academy of Hospice and Palliative Medicine, Center to Advance Palliative Care, Hospice and Palliative Nurses Association, Last Acts Partnership and the National Hospice and Palliative Care Organization.

Excerpt from the Executive Summary of the National Consensus Project for Quality Palliative Care. Reproduced with permission from the National Consensus Project for Quality Palliative Care, Pittsburgh, PA, www.nationalconsensusproject.org.

The effort to integrate palliative care into all health care for persons with debilitating and life-threatening illnesses should help to ensure that:

1. Pain and symptom control, psychosocial distress, spiritual issues, and practical needs are addressed with patient and family throughout the continuum of care.

2. Patients and families obtain the information they need in an ongoing and understandable manner, in order to grasp their condition and treatment options. Their values and goals are elicited over time; the benefits and burdens of treatment are regularly reassessed; and the decision-making process about the care plan is sensitive to changes in the patient's condition.

3. Genuine coordination of care across settings is ensured through regular and high-quality communication between providers at times of transition or changing needs, and through effective continuity of care that utilizes the techniques of case management.

4. Both patient and family are prepared for the dying process and for death, when it is anticipated. Hospice options are explored, opportunities for personal growth are enhanced and bereavement support is available for the family.

The purpose of the National Consensus Project for Quality Palliative Care is to establish Clinical Practice Guidelines that promote care of consistent and high quality, and that guide the development and structure of new and existing palliative care services. These guidelines are applicable to specialist-level palliative care delivered in a range of treatment settings, as well as to the work of providers in primary treatment settings where palliative approaches to care are integrated into daily clinical practice.

DEFINITION OF PALLIATIVE CARE

The goal of palliative care is to prevent and relieve suffering and to support the best possible quality of life for patients and their families, regardless of the stage of the disease or the need for other therapies. Palliative care is both a philosophy of care and an organized, highly structured system for delivering care. Palliative care expands traditional disease-model medical treatments to include the goals of enhancing quality of life for patient and family, optimizing function, helping with decision-making, and providing opportunities for personal growth. As such, it can be delivered concurrently with life-prolonging care or as the main focus of care.

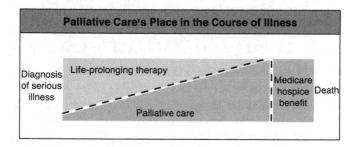

Palliative Care's Place in the Course of Illness

Diagnosis of serious illness

Life-prolonging therapy

Palliative care

Medicare hospice benefit

Death

PATIENT POPULATIONS SERVED

For the purposes of this document, the term *life-threatening or debilitating illness* is assumed to encompass the population of patients of all ages and a broad range of diagnostic categories, who are living with a persistent or recurring condition that adversely affects daily functioning or will predictably reduce life expectancy.

SPECIALTY-LEVEL PALLIATIVE CARE AND PALLIATIVE CARE IN PRIMARY TREATMENT SETTINGS

Palliative care is both a general approach to patient care that should be routinely integrated with disease-modifying therapies, and a growing practice specialty for appropriately trained physicians, nurses, social workers, chaplains, and others whose expertise is required to optimize quality of life for those with life-threatening or debilitating chronic illness. Primary practitioners, in the routine course of providing health care, are expected to provide basic elements of palliative care (e.g., pain and symptom assessment and management, advance care planning). In other cases, complexity may determine that the patient or their family requires the services of palliative care specialists. Specialist palliative care providers are professionals whose work is largely or entirely involved with palliative care and who have received appropriate training and credentialing in the field.

CORE ELEMENTS OF PALLIATIVE CARE

The National Consensus Project includes the following key elements of palliative care:

- **Patient population:** The population served includes patients of all ages experiencing a debilitating chronic or life-threatening illness, condition, or injury.

- **Patient- and family-centered care:** The uniqueness of each patient and family is respected, and the patient and family constitute the unit of care. The family is defined by the patient or, in the case of minors or those without decision-making capacity, by their surrogates. In this context, family members may be related or unrelated to the patient; they are individuals who provide support and with whom the patient has a significant relationship. The care plan is determined by the goals and preferences of the patient and family, with support and guidance in decision-making from the health care team.

- **Timing of palliative care:** Palliative care ideally begins at the time of diagnosis of a life-threatening or debilitating condition and continues through cure, or until death, and into the family's bereavement period.

- **Comprehensive care:** Palliative care employs multidimensional assessment to identify and relieve suffering through the prevention or alleviation of physical, psychological, social, and spiritual distress. Care providers should regularly assist patients and their families to understand changes in condition, and the implications of these changes as they relate to ongoing and future care and goals of treatment. Palliative care requires the regular and formal clinical process of patient-appropriate assessment, diagnosis, planning, interventions, monitoring, and follow-up.

- **Interdisciplinary team:** Palliative care presupposes indications for, and provision of, interdisciplinary team evaluation and treatment in selected cases. The palliative care team must be skilled in care of the patient population to be served. Palliative care teams may be expanded to include a range of professionals, based on the services needed. They include a core group of professionals from medicine, nursing, and social work, and may include some combination of volunteer coordinators, bereavement coordinators, chaplains, psychologists, pharmacists, nursing assistants and home attendants, dietitians, physical-, occupational-, art-, play-, child-life- and music therapists, case managers and trained volunteers.

- **Attention to relief of suffering:** The primary goal of palliative care is to prevent and relieve the many and various burdens imposed by diseases and their treatments, and consequent suffering, including pain and other symptom distress.

- **Communication skills:** Effective communication skills are requisite in palliative care. These include developmentally appropriate and effective sharing of information, active listening, determination of goals and preferences, assistance with medical decision-making, and effective communication with all individuals involved in the care of patients and their families.

- **Skill in care of the dying and the bereaved:** Palliative care specialist teams must be knowledgeable about prognostication, signs and symptoms of imminent death, and the associated care and support needs of patients and their families before and after the death, including age-specific physical and psychological syndromes, opportunities for growth, normal and aberrant grief, and bereavement processes.

- **Continuity of care across settings:** Palliative care is integral to all health care delivery system settings (hospital, emergency department, nursing home, home care, assisted living facilities, outpatient and nontraditional environments such as schools). The palliative care team collaborates with professional and informal caregivers in each of these settings, in order to ensure coordination, communication, and continuity of palliative care across institutional and home care settings. Prevention of crises and unnecessary transfers are important outcomes of palliative care.

- **Equitable access:** Palliative care teams should work toward equitable access to palliative care across all ages and patient populations, all diagnostic categories, all health care settings including rural communities, and regardless of race, ethnicity, sexual preference, or ability to pay.

- **Addressing regulatory barriers:** Concerns about drug abuse have led to increased concerns about medically appropriate use of opioid analgesics. While efforts to address abuse are necessary, they should not interfere with medical practice and the care of patients in pain. Palliative care professionals should collaborate with policy-makers, law enforcers and regulators to achieve a balanced and positive regulatory environment for pain management and palliative care.

- **Quality improvement:** Palliative care services should be committed to the pursuit of excellence and high quality of care. Determination of quality requires regular and systematic evaluation of the processes of care and measurement of outcomes data using validated instruments.

MODELS OF PALLIATIVE CARE DELIVERY

Palliative care is appropriate for all patients from the time of diagnosis with a life- threatening or debilitating condition, and service delivery should be structured accordingly. Palliative care services are most effective when integrated into specific care settings (e.g., hospital, nursing home, assisted living, home care, etc.). This requires training in the fundamentals of palliative care for practitioners in a range of primary treatment settings, as well as establishing referral patterns and access to credentialed palliative care specialists and formal palliative care teams.

Common organizational delivery models for palliative care programs inclusive of hospice programs include:

- Consultation service team (usually in a hospital, office practice setting, nursing home, or home setting), consisting of physician, nurse, and/or social work evaluations.
- Dedicated inpatient unit (acute and rehabilitation hospital, nursing home) or combined with free-standing inpatient hospice.
- Combined consultative service team and inpatient unit (hospital and nursing home).
- Combined hospice program and palliative care program (hospital, nursing home, and some freestanding hospice inpatient facilities).
- Hospital- or private-practice-based outpatient palliative care practice or clinic.
- Hospice-based palliative care at home.
- Hospice-based consultation in outpatient settings.

PALLIATIVE CARE ACROSS THE CONTINUUM

The growing need for and interest in palliative care underscores the importance of practice guidelines aimed at promoting palliative care clinical services of a high and consistent quality across all relevant care settings in the United States. Most people receive health care in multiple clinical settings: physician's offices, hospitals, school-based clinics, nursing homes, emergency facilities, and at home. It is well established that communication among these various care settings is extremely difficult, resulting in discontinuities of care. Continuity of care is especially important for patients and families facing life-threatening illness or injury. Toward this end, a core value of palliative care is the promotion and facilitation of continuity of care to avoid needless suffering and errors, eliminate patient and family perceptions of abandonment, and ensure that choices and preferences are respected.

THE NEED FOR CONSENSUS

Professional consensus on what constitutes high-quality palliative care is prerequisite to the effective delivery of such services across the continuum of care. This consensus process provides credible common ground to begin systematic improvements in palliative care delivery. In addition, the consensus process fosters the development of a broad-based and enduring palliative care constituency through the dissemination of these guidelines throughout the many sectors of the United States health care system and to policy-makers, regulators and the media.

PURPOSE OF THE CLINICAL PRACTICE GUIDELINES FOR QUALITY PALLIATIVE CARE

The mission of the National Consensus Project for Quality Palliative Care is to create a set of clinical practice guidelines to improve the quality of palliative care in the United States. Specifically, these Clinical Practice Guidelines for Quality Palliative Care aim to promote quality and reduce variation in new and existing programs, develop and encourage continuity of care across settings, and facilitate collaborative partnerships among palliative care programs, community hospices and a wide range of other health care delivery settings.

The purposes of these Clinical Practice Guidelines for Quality Palliative Care are to:

1. Facilitate the development and continuing improvement of clinical palliative care programs providing care to patients and families with life-threatening or debilitating illness.

2. Establish uniformly accepted definitions of the essential elements in palliative care that promote quality, consistency, and reliability of these services.

3. Establish national goals for access to quality palliative care.

4. Foster performance measurement and quality improvement initiatives in palliative care services.
5. Foster continuity of palliative care across settings (home, residential care, hospital, hospice).

Clinical Practice Guidelines for Quality Palliative Care

Baseline Assumptions

The following assumptions are fundamental to the development of the Clinical Practice Guidelines for Quality Palliative Care:

- **Goal guidelines:** These palliative care guidelines represent goals that palliative care services should strive to attain, as opposed to minimal or lowest acceptable practices.

- **Health care quality standards:** These palliative care guidelines assume that palliative care services will follow established practice standards and requirements for health care quality such as safety, effective leadership, medical record-keeping, and error reduction.

- **Codes of ethics:** These guidelines assume adherence to established professional and organizational codes of ethics.

- **Ongoing revision:** Palliative care guidelines will evolve as professional practice, the evidence base, and the health care system change over time. These guidelines were written assuming an ongoing process of evidence-based evaluation and revision.

- **Peer-defined guidelines:** These clinical practice guidelines were developed through a consensus process including a broad range of palliative care professionals; they are not linked to regulatory or reimbursement criteria and are not mandatory. However, they are written with the intent that they will be used as guidelines to

(Continued)

Clinical Practice Guidelines for Quality Palliative Care (*Continued*)

promote the development of highest-quality clinical palliative care services across the health care continuum.

- **Specialty care:** When this document refers to specialty-level palliative care services, it assumes provision of services by palliative care professionals within an interdisciplinary team whose work reflects substantial involvement in the care of patients with life-threatening or debilitating chronic illnesses, and their families. Palliative care qualifications are determined by organizations granting professional credentials and programmatic accreditation.

- **Continuing professional education:** These guidelines assume ongoing professional education for all palliative care professionals in the knowledge, attitudes, and skills required to deliver quality palliative care across the domains established in this document.

- **Applicability of guidelines:** These guidelines should promote integration and application of the principles, philosophy and practices of palliative care across the continuum of care by both professional and certified caregivers in these settings.

CLINICAL PRACTICE GUIDELINES FOR QUALITY PALLIATIVE CARE

Excellence in specialist-level palliative care requires expertise in the clinical management of problems in multiple domains, supported by a programmatic infrastructure that furthers the goals of care and supports practitioners. Eight domains were identified as the framework for these guidelines: Structure and Processes of Care; Physical Aspects of Care; Psychological and Psychiatric Aspects of Care; Social Aspects of Care; Spiritual,

Religious, and Existential Aspects of Care; Cultural Aspects of Care; Care of the Imminently Dying Patient; and Ethical and Legal Aspects of Care. These domains were drawn from the work of the previously established Australian, New Zealand, Canadian, Children's Hospice International and NHPCO standards efforts.

The guidelines rest on fundamental processes that cross all domains and encompass assessment, information sharing, decision-making, care planning, and care delivery. Each domain is followed by specific clinical practice guidelines regarding professional behavior and service delivery. These are followed by justifications, supporting and clarifying statements, and suggested criteria for assessing whether or not the identified expectation has been met. References to the literature supporting these recommendations are included in the guidelines.

Domains of Quality Palliative Care

1. Structure and Processes of Care

2. Physical Aspects of Care

3. Psychological and Psychiatric Aspects of Care

4. Social Aspects of Care

5. Spiritual, Religious, and Existential Aspects of Care

6. Cultural Aspects of Care

7. Care of the Imminently Dying Patient

8. Ethical and Legal Aspects of Care

DOMAIN 1: STRUCTURE AND PROCESSES OF CARE[22-34]

Guideline 1.1 The plan of care is based on a comprehensive interdisciplinary assessment of the patient and family

Criteria:

- Assessment and its documentation are interdisciplinary and coordinated.
- Initial and subsequent assessments are carried out through patient and family interview, review of medical records, discussion with other providers, physical examination and assessment, and relevant laboratory and/or diagnostic tests or procedures.
- Assessment includes documentation of disease status, including diagnoses and prognosis; co-morbid medical and psychiatric disorders; physical and psychological symptoms; functional status; social, cultural, spiritual and advance care planning concerns and preferences, including appropriateness of referral to hospice. Assessment of children must be conducted with consideration of age and stage of neurocognitive development.
- Patient and family expectations, goals for care and for living, understanding of the disease and prognosis, as well as preferences for the type and site of care are assessed and documented.
- The assessment is reviewed on a regular basis.

Guideline 1.2 The care plan is based on the identified and expressed values, goals and needs of patient and family, and is developed with professional guidance and support for decision-making

Criteria:

- The care plan is based upon an ongoing assessment, determined by goals set with patient and family, and with consideration of the changing benefit/burden assessment at critical decision points during the course of illness.

- The care plan is developed through the input of patient, family, caregivers, involved health care providers, and the palliative care team with the additional input, when indicated, of other specialists and caregivers, such as school professionals, clergy, friends, etc.
- Care plan changes are based on the evolving needs and preferences of the patient and family over time, and recognize the complex, competing, and shifting priorities in goals of care.
- The interdisciplinary team coordinates and shares the information, provides support for decision-making, develops and carries out the care plan, and communicates the palliative care plan to patient and family, to all involved health professionals and to the responsible providers when patients transfer to different care settings.
- Treatment and care setting alternatives are clearly documented and communicated, and permit the patient and their family to make informed choices.
- Treatment decisions are based on goals of care, assessment of risk and benefit, best evidence, and patient/family preferences. Re-evaluation of treatment efficacy and patient-family preferences is documented.
- The evolving care plan must be clearly documented over time.

Guideline 1.3 An interdisciplinary team provides services to the patient and family, consistent with the care plan

Criteria:

- Specialist-level palliative care is delivered by an interdisciplinary team.
- The team includes palliative care professionals with the appropriate patient population-specific education, credentialing and experience, and ability to meet physical, psychological, social

and spiritual needs of the patient and their family. Of particular importance is hiring physicians, nurses, and social workers appropriately trained and ultimately certified in hospice and palliative care.

- The interdisciplinary palliative care team involved in the care of children, either as patients or the children of adult patients, has expertise in the delivery of services for such children.
- The patient and family have access to palliative care expertise and staff 24 hours per day, 7 days per week.
- Respite services are available for the families and caregivers of children or adults with life-threatening illnesses.
- The interdisciplinary team communicates regularly (at least weekly, more often as required by the clinical situation) to plan, review, and evaluate the care plan, with input from both patient and family.
- The team meets regularly to discuss provision of quality care, including staffing, policies, and clinical practices.
- Team leadership has appropriate training, qualifications and experience.
- Policies for prioritizing and responding to referrals in a timely manner are documented.

Guideline 1.4 The interdisciplinary team may include appropriately trained and supervised volunteers

Criteria:

- If volunteers participate, policies and procedures are in place to ensure the necessary education of volunteers, and to guide recruitment, screening, training, work practices, support, supervision, and performance evaluation, and to clarify the responsibilities of the program to its volunteers.
- Volunteers are screened, educated, coordinated, and supervised by an appropriately educated and experienced professional team member.

Guideline 1.5 Support for education and training is available to the interdisciplinary team

Criteria:

* Educational resources and continuing professional education focused on the domains of palliative care contained in this document are regularly provided to staff, and participation is documented.

Guideline 1.6 The palliative care program is committed to quality improvement in clinical and management practices

Criteria:

* The palliative care program must be committed to the pursuit of excellence and highest quality of care and support for all patients and their families. Determining quality requires regular and systematic measurement, analysis, review, evaluation, goal setting, and revision of the processes and outcomes of care provided by the program.
* Quality care must incorporate attention at all times to:
  — Safety, and the systems of care that reduce error.
  — Timeliness, care delivered to the right patient at the right time.
  — Patient-centered care, based on the goals and preferences of the patient and the family.
  — Beneficial and/or effective care, demonstrably influencing important patient outcomes or processes of care linked to desirable outcomes.
  — Equity, care that is available to all in need and who could benefit.
  — Efficiency, care designed to meet the actual needs of the patient so that it does not waste resources.
* The palliative care program establishes quality improvement policies and procedures.
* Quality improvement activities are routine, regular and reported, and are shown to influence clinical practice.

- The clinical practices of palliative care programs reflect the integration and dissemination of research and evidence of quality improvement.
- Quality improvement activities for clinical services are collaborative, interdisciplinary, and focused on meeting the identified needs of patients and their families.
- Patients, families, health professionals, and the community may provide input for evaluation of the program.

Guideline 1.7 The palliative care program recognizes the emotional impact on the palliative care team of providing care to patients with life-threatening illnesses and their families

Criteria:

- Emotional support is available to staff and volunteers as appropriate.
- Policies guide the support of staff and volunteers, including regular meetings for review and discussion of the impact and processes of providing palliative care.

Guideline 1.8 Palliative care programs should have a relationship with one or more hospices and other community resources in order to ensure continuity of the highest-quality palliative care across the illness trajectory

Criteria:

- Palliative care programs must support and promote continuity of care across settings and throughout the trajectory of illness.
- As appropriate, patients and families are routinely informed about and offered referral to hospice and other community-based health care resources.

- Referring physicians and health care providers are routinely informed about the availability and benefits of hospice and other community resources for care for their patients and families, as appropriate and indicated.

- Policies for formal written and verbal communication about all domains in the plan of care are established between the palliative care program, hospice programs and other major community providers involved in the patients' care. Policies enable timely and effective sharing of information among teams while safeguarding privacy.

- Where possible, hospice and palliative care program staff routinely participate in each other's team meetings to promote regular professional communication, collaboration and an integrated plan of care on behalf of patients and families.

- Palliative care and hospice care programs, as well as other major community providers, routinely seek opportunities to collaborate and work in partnership to promote increased access to quality palliative care across the continuum.

Guideline 1.9 The physical environment in which care is provided should meet the preferences, needs and circumstances of the patient and family to the extent possible

Criteria:

- When feasible, care is provided in the setting preferred by the patient and their family.

- When care is provided away from the patient's home, the care setting addresses safety and, as appropriate and feasible, flexible and open visiting hours, space for families to visit, rest, eat, or prepare meals, and meet with the palliative care team and other professionals, as well as privacy and other needs identified by the family. The setting should address the unique care needs of children as patients, family members, or visitors.

DOMAIN 2: PHYSICAL ASPECTS OF CARE[35-56]

Guideline 2.1 Pain, other symptoms and side effects are managed based upon the best available evidence, which is skillfully and systematically applied

Criteria:

- The interdisciplinary team includes professionals with specialist-level skill in symptom control.

- Regular, ongoing assessment of pain, nonpain symptoms (including but not limited to shortness of breath, nausea, fatigue and weakness, anorexia, insomnia, anxiety, depression, confusion, and constipation), treatment of side effects, and functional capacities are documented. Validated instruments, where available, should be used. Symptom assessment in children and cognitively impaired patients should be performed with appropriate tools.

- The outcome of pain and symptom management is the safe and timely reduction of pain and symptom levels, for as long as the symptom persists, to a level that is acceptable to the patient.

- Response to symptom distress is prompt and tracked, through documentation in the medical record.

- Barriers to effective pain management should be recognized and addressed, including inappropriate fears of the risks of side effects, addiction, respiratory depression, and hastening of death in association with opioid analgesics.

- A risk management plan should be implemented when controlled substances are prescribed for long-term symptom management.

- Patient understanding of disease and its consequences, symptoms, side effects of treatments, functional impairment and potentially useful treatments is assessed. The capacity of the patient to secure and accept needed care and to cope with the illness and its consequences is assessed.

- Family understanding of the disease and its consequences, symptoms, side effects, functional impairment and treatments is assessed. The capacity of the family to secure and provide needed care and to cope with the illness and its consequences is assessed.

- Treatment of distressing symptoms and side effects incorporates pharmacological, nonpharmacological, and complementary/supportive therapies. Approach to the relief of suffering is comprehensive, addressing physical, psychological, social, and spiritual aspects.

- Referrals to health care professionals with specialized skills in symptom management are made available when appropriate (e.g., radiation therapists, anesthesia pain management specialists, orthopedists, physical and occupational therapists, and child-life specialists).

- Family is educated and supported to provide safe and appropriate comfort measures to the patient. Family is provided with backup resources for response to urgent needs.

- A process for quality improvement and review of physical and functional assessment and effectiveness of treatment is documented and leads to change in clinical practice.

DOMAIN 3: PSYCHOLOGICAL AND PSYCHIATRIC ASPECTS OF CARE[30,57–73]

Guideline 3.1 Psychological and psychiatric issues are assessed and managed based upon the best available evidence, which is skillfully and systematically applied

Criteria:

- The interdisciplinary team includes professionals with patient-specific skill and training in the psychological consequences and psychiatric co-morbidities of serious illness for both patient and family, including depression, anxiety, delirium, and cognitive impairment.

- Regular, ongoing assessment of psychological reactions (including but not limited to stress, anticipatory grieving and coping strategies) and psychiatric conditions occurs and is documented. Whenever possible, a validated and context-specific assessment tool should be used.
- Psychological assessment includes patient understanding of disease, symptoms, side effects and their treatments, as well as assessment of care giving needs, capacity, and coping strategies.
- Psychological assessment includes family understanding of the illness and its consequences for the patient as well as the family, and the assessment of family caregiving capacities, needs, and coping strategies.
- Family is educated and supported to provide safe and appropriate psychological support measures to the patient.
- Pharmacologic, nonpharmacologic, and complementary therapies are employed in the treatment of psychological distress or psychiatric syndromes, as appropriate. Treatment alternatives are clearly documented and communicated, and permit the patient and family to make informed choices.
- Response to symptom distress is prompt and tracked through documentation in the medical record. Regular re-evaluation of treatment efficacy and patient-family preferences is documented.
- Referrals to health care professionals with specialized skills in age-appropriate psychological and psychiatric management are made available when appropriate (e.g., psychiatrists, psychologists, and social workers). Identified psychiatric co-morbidities in family or caregivers are referred for treatment.
- Developmentally appropriate assessment and support are provided to pediatric patients, their siblings, and the children or grandchildren of adult patients.
- Communication with children and cognitively impaired individuals occurs using verbal, nonverbal, and/or symbolic means appropriate to developmental stage and cognitive capacity.

- Treatment decisions are based on goals of care, assessment of risk and benefit, best evidence, and patient/family preferences. The goal is to address psychological needs, treat psychiatric disorders, promote adjustment, and support opportunities for emotional growth, healing, reframing, completion of unfinished business, and support through the bereavement period.
- A process for quality improvement and review of psychological and psychiatric assessment and effectiveness of treatment is documented and leads to change in clinical practice.

Guideline 3.2 A grief and bereavement program is available to patients and families, based on the assessed need for services

Criteria:

- The interdisciplinary team includes professionals with patient-population-appropriate education and skill in the care of patients and families experiencing loss, grief, and bereavement.
- Bereavement services are recognized as a core component of the palliative care program.
- Bereavement services and follow-up are made available to the family for at least 12 months, or as long as is needed, after the death of the patient.
- Grief and bereavement risk assessment is routine, developmentally appropriate and ongoing for the patient and family throughout the illness trajectory, recognizing issues of loss and grief in living with a life-threatening illness.
- Clinical assessment is used to identify people at risk of complicated grief and bereavement, and its association with depression and co-morbid complications, particularly among the elderly.
- Information on loss and grief and the availability of bereavement support services, including those available through hospice and other community programs, is made routinely

available to families before and after the death of the patient, as culturally appropriate and desired.

- Support and grief interventions are provided in accordance with developmental, cultural and spiritual needs, expectations and preferences of the family, including attention to the needs of siblings of pediatric patients and children of adult patients.
- Staff and volunteers who provide bereavement services receive ongoing education, supervision and support.
- Referrals to health care professionals with specialized skills are made when clinically indicated.

DOMAIN 4: SOCIAL ASPECTS OF CARE[74–83]

Guideline 4.1 Comprehensive interdisciplinary assessment identifies the social needs of patients and their families, and a care plan is developed in order to respond to these needs as effectively as possible

Criteria:
- The interdisciplinary team includes professionals with patient-population-specific skills in the assessment and management of social and practical needs during a life-threatening or chronic debilitating illness.
- Practitioners skilled in the assessment and management of the developmental needs of children should be available for pediatric patients and the children of adult patients, as appropriate.
- A comprehensive interdisciplinary social assessment is completed and documented to include: family structure and geographic location; relationships; lines of communication; existing social and cultural network; perceived social support;

medical decision-making; work and school settings; finances; sexuality; intimacy; living arrangements; caregiver availability; access to transportation; access to prescription and over-the-counter medicines and nutritional products; access to needed equipment; community resources including school and work settings; and legal issues. Routine patient and family meetings are conducted with members of the interdisciplinary team to assess understanding and address questions; provide information and help with decision-making; discuss goals of care and advance care planning; determine wishes, preferences, hopes, and fears; provide emotional and social support; and enhance communication.

- The social care plan is formulated from a comprehensive social and cultural assessment and reassessment, and reflects and documents values, goals, and preferences as set by patient and family over time. Interventions are planned to minimize adverse impact of caregiving on the family and to promote caregiver and family goals and well-being.

- Referrals to appropriate services are made that meet identified social needs and promote access to care, help in the home, school or work, transportation, rehabilitation, medications, counseling, community resources, and equipment.

DOMAIN 5: SPIRITUAL, RELIGIOUS AND EXISTENTIAL ASPECTS OF CARE[84–92]

Guideline 5.1 Spiritual and existential dimensions are assessed and responded to based upon the best available evidence, which is skillfully and systematically applied

Criteria:

- The interdisciplinary team includes professionals with skill in assessing and responding to the spiritual and existential issues that pediatric and adult patients with life-threatening illnesses and conditions, and their families, are likely to confront.

- Regular, ongoing exploration of spiritual and existential concerns occurs and is documented (including but not limited to life review, assessment of hopes and fears, meaning, purpose, beliefs about afterlife, guilt, forgiveness, and life completion tasks). Whenever possible, a standardized instrument should be used.
- A spiritual assessment is utilized to identify religious or spiritual/ existential background, preferences and related beliefs, rituals, and practices of the patient and family.
- Periodic re-evaluation of the impact of spiritual/existential interventions and patient-family preferences is documented.
- Spiritual/existential care needs, goals, and concerns are addressed and documented, and support is offered for issues of life completion in a manner consistent with the individual's and family's cultural and religious values.
- Pastoral care and other palliative care professionals facilitate contacts with spiritual/religious communities, groups, or individuals, as desired by the patient and/or family, and patients have access to clergy in their own religious traditions.
- Professional and institutional use of religious symbols is sensitive to cultural and religious diversity.
- The patient and family are encouraged to display their own religious/spiritual symbols.
- The palliative care service facilitates religious or spiritual rituals as desired by patient and family, especially at the time of death.
- Referrals to professionals with specialized knowledge or skills in spiritual and existential issues are made available when appropriate (e.g., to a chaplain familiar with or from the patient's own religious tradition).
- A process for quality improvement is documented and leads to change in clinical practice.

DOMAIN 6: CULTURAL ASPECTS OF CARE[77,80,87,93-101]

Guideline 6.1 The palliative care program assesses and attempts to meet the culture-specific needs of the patient and family

Criteria:

- The cultural background, concerns, and needs of the patient and their family are elicited and documented.
- Cultural needs identified by team and family are addressed in the interdisciplinary team care plan.
- Communication with patient and family is respectful of their cultural preferences regarding disclosure, truth-telling, and decision-making.
- The program aims to respect and accommodate the range of language, dietary, and ritual practices of the patients and their families.
- When possible, the team has access to and utilizes appropriate interpreter services.
- Recruitment and hiring practices strive to reflect the cultural diversity of the community.

DOMAIN 7: CARE OF THE IMMINENTLY DYING PATIENT[102-107]

Guideline 7.1 Signs and symptoms of impending death are recognized and communicated, and care appropriate for this phase of illness is provided to patient and family

Criteria:

- The patient's and family's transition to the actively dying phase is recognized, when possible, and is documented and communicated appropriately to patient, family, and staff.

- End-of-life concerns, hopes, fears, and expectations are addressed openly and honestly in the context of social and cultural customs in a developmentally appropriate manner.
- Symptoms at the end of life are assessed and documented with appropriate frequency and are treated based on patient-family preferences.
- The care plan is revised to meet the unique needs of the patient and family at this phase of the illness. The need for higher intensity and acuity of care during the active dying phase is met and documented.
- Patient and family wishes regarding care setting for the death are documented. Any inability to meet these needs and preferences is reviewed and addressed by the palliative care team.
- As patients decline, the hospice referral option will be introduced (or reintroduced) for those who have not accessed hospice services.
- The family is educated regarding the signs and symptoms of approaching death in a developmentally, culturally, and age-appropriate manner.

DOMAIN 8: ETHICAL AND LEGAL ASPECTS OF CARE [108–123]

Guideline 8.1 The patient's goals, preferences, and choices are respected within the limits of applicable state and federal law, and form the basis for the plan of care

Criteria:

- The interdisciplinary team includes professionals with knowledge and skill in ethical, legal, and regulatory aspects of medical decision-making.
- The patient's or surrogate's expressed wishes, in collaboration with the family and the interdisciplinary team, form the basis for the care plan.

- The adult patient with decisional capacity determines the level of involvement of the family in decision-making and communication about the care plan.

- Evidence of patient preferences for care is routinely sought and documented in the medical record. Failure to honor these preferences is documented and addressed by the team.

- Among minors with decision-making capacity, the child's views and preferences for medical care, including assent for treatment, should be documented and given appropriate weight in decision-making. When the child's wishes differ from those of the adult decision-maker, appropriate professional staff members are available to assist the child.

- The palliative care program promotes advance care planning in order to understand and communicate the patient's or appropriate surrogate's preferences for care across the health care continuum.

- When patients are unable to communicate, the palliative care program seeks to identify advance care directives, evidence of previously expressed wishes, values, and preferences, and the appropriate surrogate decision-makers. The team must advocate the observance of previously expressed wishes of patient or surrogate, when necessary.

- Assistance is provided to surrogate decision-makers on the legal and ethical bases for surrogate decision-making, including honoring the patient's known preferences, substituted judgment and best interest criteria.

Guideline 8.2 The palliative care program is aware of and addresses the complex ethical issues arising in the care of persons with life-threatening debilitating illness

Criteria:

- Ethical concerns commonly encountered in palliative care are recognized and addressed, using ethical principles to prevent or resolve ethical dilemmas, including: beneficence; respect for persons and self-determination and associated regulatory requirements for truth-telling; capacity assessment; confidentiality; assent and permission for persons not of legal age to consent; informed consent; attention to justice and non-maleficence and associated avoidance of conflicts of interest. The team recognizes the role of cultural variation in the application of professional obligations, including truth-telling, disclosure, decisional authority, and decisions to forego therapy. Attention must be paid to the role of children and adolescents in decision-making.

- Care is consistent with the professional codes of ethics, and the scope, standards, and code of ethics of palliative care practice are modeled on existing professional codes of ethics for all relevant disciplines.

- The palliative care team aims to prevent, identify and resolve ethical dilemmas related to specific interventions, such as withholding or withdrawing treatments (including nutrition and hydration), instituting DNR orders and the use of sedation in palliative care.

- Ethical issues are documented; referrals are made to ethics consultants or committee, as appropriate.

Guideline 8.3 The palliative care program is knowledgeable about legal and regulatory aspects of palliative care

Criteria:

- Palliative care practitioners are knowledgeable about legal and regulatory issues, including federal and state statutes and regulations regarding medical decision-making, advance care planning and directives, the roles and responsibilities of surrogate decision-makers; barriers to pain relief, the legal requirements for use of controlled substances and the imperative that regulatory policy not interfere with patient care; pronouncing death; request for autopsy and organ transplant; and associated documentation in the medical record.

- Patients and families are routinely advised of the need to seek professional advice on creating or updating property wills and guardianship agreements.

CONCLUSION

Palliative care services aim to support patients of all ages with debilitating and life-threatening illness, and their families, through the full course of illness, regardless of its duration, until cure or until death, and through the bereavement period. Palliative care is delivered through skilled and interdisciplinary attention to pain and other distressing symptoms; emotional, spiritual, and practical support; assistance with complex medical decision-making; and coordination across the continuum of health care settings. The goal is to help the patient and family achieve the best possible quality of life in accordance with their values, needs, and preferences. These guidelines for quality palliative care programs represent a consensus opinion of the major palliative care organizations and leaders in the United States, and are based both on the available scientific evidence and expert professional opinion.

Clinical practice guidelines such as these have become the accepted means of promoting consistency, comprehensiveness, and quality across many domains of health care. The widespread adoption of these guidelines in the United States will help to establish palliative care as an integral component of the health care of persons living with life-threatening and debilitating chronic illness. It is hoped that the Clinical Practice Guidelines for Quality Palliative Care will encourage access to high quality palliative care that patients and families can come to expect and rely upon.

REFERENCES

1. American Academy of Pediatrics, Committee on Bioethics and Committee on Hospital Care: Palliative care for children. *Pediatrics* 2000;106(2 Pt 1):351–357.
2. American Association of Colleges of Nursing: Peaceful Death: Recommended Competencies and Curricular Guidelines for

End-of-Life Nursing Care. Washington, D.C.: American Association of Colleges of Nursing, 2002. Available at www.aacn. nche.edu/Publications/deathfin.htm.

3. American Board of Internal Medicine Committee on Evaluation of Clinical Competence: Caring for the Dying: Identification and Promotion of Physician Competency. Philadelphia: American Board of Internal Medicine, 1998.

4. American College of Surgeons: The American College of Surgeons statement on principles guiding care at the end of life. *J Am Coll Surg* 2002;194(5):664.

5. American Geriatrics Society Ethics Committee: The care of dying patients: a position statement from the American Geriatrics Society. *J Am Geriatr Soc* 1994;43(5):577–578. Available at www.americangeriatrics.org/products/positionpa-pers/ careofd.shtml.

6. American Society of Clinical Oncology End of Life Task Force: Cancer care during the last phase of life. *J Clin Oncol* 1998;16: 1986–1996.

7. Association for Palliative Medicine of Great Britain and Ireland: Curriculum for Higher Specialist Training in Palliative Medicine (2001) and Detailed Competencies for Higher Specialist Training in Palliative Medicine (2002). Southampton, Great Britain: Association for Palliative Medicine of Great Britain and Ireland. Available at www.palliative-medicine.org. [Contact sheilarichards@btconnect.com]

8. Cassel CK, Field MJ, (eds): Approaching Death: Improving Care at the End of Life. Washington, D.C.: Institute of Medicine, National Academy Press, 1997.

9. Children's International Project on Palliative/Hospice Services (ChIPPS): A Call For Change: Recommendations to Improve the Care of Children Living with Life-Threatening conditions. Alexandria, VA., 2001. Available at www. nhpco.org.

10. Drug Enforcement Administration: Promoting Pain Relief and Preventing Abuse of Pain Medications: A Critical Balancing Act. A Joint Statement from 21 Health Organizations and the Drug Enforcement Administration. Washington, D.C.: Last Acts, 2001. Available at www.medsch.wisc.edu/painpolicy/ dea01.htm.

11. Ferris FD, Balfour HM, Bowen K, Farley J, Hardwick M, Lamontagne C, Lundy M, Syme A, West P: A Model Guide to Hospice palliative care: based on national principles and norms of practice. Ottawa: Canadian Hospice Palliative Care Association, 2002. Available at www.chpca.net/publications/norms_of_practice.htm.

12. Field MJ, Behrman DE, (eds): *When Children Die: Improving Palliative and End-of-Life Care for Children and Their Families.* Washington, D.C.: Institute of Medicine, National Academy Press, 2003.

13. Hospice and Palliative Nurses Association, American Nurses Association: *Scope and Standards of Hospice and Palliative Nursing Practice.* Washington, D.C.: American Nurses Publishing, 2002.

14. Institute of Medicine Committee on Quality of Health Care in America: *Crossing the Quality Chasm.* Washington D.C.: Institute of Medicine, National Academy Press, 2001.

15. Jennings B, Ryndes T, D'Onofrio C, Baily, MA: Access to Hospice Care: Expanding Boundaries, Overcoming Barriers. Hastings Cent Rep 2003; Suppl.33(2):S1–59.

16. Last Acts: Means to a Better End: A Report on Dying in America Today. Washington, D.C.: Last Acts 2002. Available at www.lastacts.org.

17. National Hospice and Palliative Care Organization: Standards of Practice for Hospice Programs. Alexandria, VA: National Hospice and Palliative Care Organization, 2000. Available at www.nhpco.org.

18. National Hospice and Palliative Care Organization: NHPCO Facts and Figures. Alexandria, VA: National Hospice and Palliative Care Organization, 2004. Available at www.nhpco.org/files/public/Facts%20Figures%20Feb04.pdf.

19. Palliative Care Australia: Standards for Palliative Care Provision—Third Edition, 1999. Available at www.pallcare.org.au/publications/Standards_99.pdf.

20. Schapiro R, Byock I: Living and Dying Well with Cancer: Successfully Integrating Palliative Care and Cancer Treatment. Princeton, NJ: Promoting Excellence in the End of Life, Robert Wood Johnson Foundation, 2003.

21. Teno J: TIME: Toolkit of Instruments to Measure End-of-Life Care. Providence, RI: Center for Gerontology and Health Care Research, Brown Medical School, 2000. Available at www.chcr. brown.edu/pcoc/toolkit.htm.

22. Doyle D (ed): *Volunteers in Hospice and Palliative Care: A Handbook for Volunteer Service Managers*. New York: Oxford University Press, 2003.

23. Emanuel LL, von Gunten CF, Ferris FD: Education for Physicians on End-of-Life Care (EPEC) Curriculum. Chicago: American Medical Association, 1999. Available at www.ama-assn. org/ama/pub/category/2910.html.

24. Kristjanson LJ: Indicators of quality of palliative care from a family perspective. *J Palliat Care*. 1986;1(2):8–17.

25. Lickiss JN, Turner KS, Pollock MS: The interdisciplinary team. In: Doyle D, Hanks G, Cherny N, Calman K (eds): *Oxford Textbook of Palliative Medicine*. Oxford: Oxford University Press, 2004:42–46.

26. Lo B, Quill T, Tulsky J for the ACP-ASIM End-of-Life Care Consensus Panel: Discussing palliative care with patients. *Ann Intern Med* 1999;130(9):744–749.

27. Meier DE, Back AL, Morrison RS: The inner life of physicians and care of the seriously ill. *JAMA* 2001;286(23):3007–3014.

28. Monroe B. Social work in palliative medicine. In: Doyle D, Hanks G, Cherny N, Calman K (eds): *Oxford Textbook of Palliative Medicine*. Oxford: Oxford University Press, 2004: 1005–1017.

29. Quill TE: Perspectives on care at the close of life. Initiating end-of-life discussions with seriously ill patients: addressing the elephant in the room. *JAMA*. 2000;284(19):2502–2507.

30. Singer PA, Martin DK, Kelner M, Marm M: Domains of quality end-of-life care from the patients' perspective. *JAMA*. 1999;281: 162–168.

31. Steinhauser KE, Christakis NA, Clipp EC, McNeilly M, McIntyre L, Tulsky JA: Factors considered important at the end of life by patients, family, physicians, and other care providers. *JAMA*. 2000;284:2476–2482.

32. SUPPORT Principal Investigators: A controlled trial to improve care for seriously ill hospitalized patients. The study

to understand prognoses and preferences for outcomes and risks of treatments (SUPPORT). *JAMA*. 1995;274:1591–1598.

33. Vachon M: Caring for the caregiver in oncology and palliative care. *Semin Oncol Nurs*. 1998;14(2):152–157.

34. Zwarenstein M, Reeves S, Barr H, Hammick M, Koppel I, Atkins J: Interprofessional education: effects on professional practice and health care outcomes. *Cochrane Database Syst Rev*. 2001;(1):CD002213.

35. American Geriatrics Society: The management of chronic pain in older persons. *J Am Geriatr Soc* 1998;46(5):635–651.

36. American Pain Society Quality of Care Committee: Quality improvement guidelines for the treatment of acute pain and cancer pain. *JAMA*. 1995;274:1874–1880.

37. Benedetti CC, Brock C, Berger AM, Cleeland C, Coyle N, Dube JE, Ferrell B, Hassenbusch S 3rd, Janjan NA, Lema MJ, Levy MH, Loscalzo MJ, Lynch M, Muir C, Oakes L, O'Neill A, Payne R, Syrjala KL, Urba S, Weinstein SM: National Comprehensive Cancer Network. Practice Guidelines for Cancer Pain. *Oncology* (Huntington) 2000;14(11A):135–150.

38. Ben-Zacharia B, Lublin FD: Palliative care in patients with multiple sclerosis. *Neurol Clin*. 2001;19(4):801–827.

39. Ferrell BR, Coyle N, (eds): *Textbook of Palliative Nursing*. New York: Oxford University Press, 2001.

40. Borasio GD, Shaw PJ, Hardiman O, Ludolph AC, Sales Luis ML, Silani V for the European ALS Study Group: Standards of palliative care for patients with amyotrophic lateral sclerosis: results of a European survey. *Amyotroph Lateral Scler Other Motor Neuron Disord* 2001;2:159–164.

41. Breitbart, W, Chochinov H, Passik S: Psychiatric aspect of palliative care. In: Doyle DD, Hanks WC, McDonald N (eds):. *Oxford Textbook of Palliative Medicine*, 2nd ed. New York: Oxford University Press, 1998:933–959.

42. Bruera E, Portenoy R, (eds): *Topics in Palliative Care*, Volume 2. New York: Oxford University Press, 1998.

43. Bruera E, Portenoy R, (eds). *Topics in Palliative Care*, Volume 5. New York: Oxford University Press, 2001.

44. Chang VH, Thaler HT, Polyak TA, Kornblith AB, Lepore JM, Portenoy RK: Quality of life and survival: the role of

multidimensional symptom assessment. Cancer 1998;83(1): 173–179.

45. Doyle, D., Hanks G.W.C., Cherny N, Calman K, (eds): *Oxford Textbook of Palliative Medicine*, 3rd ed. New York, NY: Oxford University Press, 2004.

46. Ferrell BR, Bendnash G, Grant M, Rhome A: End of Life Nursing Consortium (ELNEC), 2000. Available at www.aacn. nche.edu/elnec.

47. Greenberg BR, McCorkle R, Vlahov D, Selwyn PA: Palliative care for HIV disease in the era of highly active antiretroviral therapy. J Urban Health 2000;77:150–165.

48. Hodson ME: Treatment of cystic fibrosis in the adult. Respiration 2000;67(6):595–607.

49. Lynn J, Ely W, Zhong G, NcNiff KL, Dawson NV, Connors A, Desbiens NA, Claessens M, McCarthy EP: Living and dying with chronic obstructive pulmonary disease. *J Am Geriatr Soc* 2000; 48(5 Suppl):S91–S100.

50. McCaffery M, Pasero C: *Pain Clinical Manual*. St. Louis, Missouri: Mosby, 1999.

51. Persons A: The management of persistent pain in older persons. *J Am Geriatr Soc.* 2002;50(6 Suppl):S205–224.

52. Portenoy R, Bruera E (eds): *Topics in Palliative Care*, Volume 1. New York: Oxford University Press, 1997.

53. Portenoy R, Bruera E (eds): *Topics in Palliative Care*, Volume 3. New York: Oxford University Press, 1998.

54. Portenoy R, Bruera E (eds): *Topics in Palliative Care*, Volume 4. New York: Oxford University Press, 2000.

55. Wilkie DJ, Brown MA, Corless I, Farber S, Judge K, Shannon S, Wells MJ: Toolkit for Nursing Excellence at End-of-Life Transition. Seattle: The Robert Wood Johnson Foundation 2001: CD-ROM.

56. Wolfe J, Grier HE, Klar N, Levin SB, Ellenbogen JM, Ellenbogen JM, Salem-Schatz S, Emanuel EJ, Weeks JC: Symptoms and suffering at the end of life in children with cancer. *N Engl J Med.* 2000;342:326–333.

57. American Academy of Pediatrics: The pediatrician and childhood bereavement. *Pediatrics.* 2000;105(2):445–447.

58. Bouton BL: The interdisciplinary bereavement team: defining and directing appropriate bereavement care. *Hosp J.* 1996; 11(4):15–24.

59. Brown CK: Bereavement care. Br J Gen Pract 1995;45(395):327.

60. Casarett D, Kutner JS, Abrahm J for the End-of-Life Consensus Panel: Life after death: a practical approach to grief and bereavement. *Ann Intern Med.* 2001;134(3):208–215.

61. Chochinov HM, Hack T, McClement S, Kristjanson L, Harlos M: Dignity in the terminally ill: a developing empirical model *Soc Sci Med.* 2002;54(3):433–443.

62. Cohen SR, Leis A: What determines the quality of life of terminally ill cancer patients from their own perspective? *J Palliat Care.* 2002;18(1):48–58.

63. Gillance H, Tucker A.,Aldridge J, Wright JB: Bereavement: providing support for siblings. *Paediatr Nurs.* 1997;9(5):22–24.

64. Hockley J: Psychosocial aspects in palliative care—communicating with the patient and family. *Acta Oncologica.* 2000;39(8):905–910.

65. Maddocks I: Grief and bereavement. Med J Aust 2003;179 (6 Suppl): S6–7.

66. Main J: Management of relatives of patients who are dying. *J Clin Nurs.* 2002;11(6):794–801.

67. Prigerson HG, Jacobs SC: Perspectives on care at the close of life. Caring for bereaved patients: "All the doctors just suddenly go." *JAMA.* 2001;286(11):1369–1376.

68. Rando TA: *Treatment of Complicated Grief.* Champaign, IL: Research Press, 1993.

69. Rando TA (ed): *Clinical Dimension of Anticipatory Mourning.* Champaign, IL: Research Press, 2000.

70. Teno JM: Putting patient and family voice back into measuring quality of care for the dying. *Hosp J.* 1999;14(3–4):167–176.

71. Vachon ML, Kristjanson L, Higginson I: Psychosocial issues in palliative care: the patient, the family, and the process and outcome of care. *J Pain Symptom Manage.* 1995;10(2): 142–150.

72. Vachon, MLS: The stress of professional caregivers. In: Doyle D, Hanks GW, Cherny N, Calman K, (eds): *Oxford Textbook of*

Palliative Medicine, 3rd ed. Oxford: Oxford University Press, 2004:992–1004.

73. Werth JL Jr, Gordon JR, Johnson RR Jr: Psychosocial issues near the end of life. *Aging Ment Health*. 2002;6(4):402–412.

74. Baluss ME: Palliative care: ethics and the law. In: Berger A, Portenoy RK, Weissman DE, (eds): *Principles and Practice of Palliative Care and Supportive Oncology*, 2nd ed. Philadelphia: Lippincott Williams & Wilkins, 2002:902–914.

75. Covinsky KE, Goldman L, Cook EF, Oye R, Desbiens N, Reding D, Fulkerson W, Connors AF Jr, Lynn J, Phillips RS: The impact of serious illness on patients' families. SUPPORT Investigators. Study to Understand Prognoses and Preferences for Outcomes and Risks of Treatment. *JAMA*. 1994;272(23):1839–1844.

76. Covinsky KE, Landefeld CS, Teno J, Connors AF Jr, Dawson N, Youngner S, Desbiens N, Lynn J, Fulkerson W, Reding D, Oye R, Phillips RS: Is economic hardship on the families of the seriously ill associated with patient and surrogate care preferences? SUPPORT Investigators. Arch Intern Med 1996;156(15):1737–1741.

77. Crawley LM, Marshall PA, Lo B, Koenig BA for the End-of-Life Care Consensus Panel: Strategies for culturally effective end-of-life care. *Ann Intern Med*. 2002;136(9):673–679.

78. Curtis JR, Patrick DL, Shannon SE, Treece PD, Engelberg RA, Rubenfeld GD: The family conference as a focus to improve communication about end-of-life care in the intensive care unit: opportunities for improvement. *Crit Care Med*. 2001; 29(2 Suppl):N26–33.

79. Emanuel EJ, Fairclough DL, Slutsman J, Emanuel LL: Understanding economic and other burdens of terminal illness: the experience of patients and their caregivers. *Ann Intern Med*. 2000;132(6):451–459.

80. Koenig BA, Gates-Williams J: Understanding cultural difference in caring for dying patients. *West J Med*. 1995;163(3):244–249.

81. Rice AM: Sexuality in cancer and palliative care 1: Effects of disease and treatment. *Int J Palliat Nurs*. 2000;6(8):392–397.

82. Rice AM: Sexuality in cancer and palliative care 2: Exploring the issues. *Int J Palliat Nurs*. 2000;6(9):448–453.

83. Scott JT, Harmsen M, Prictor MJ, Sowden AJ, Watt I: Interventions for improving communication with children and adolescents about their cancer. Cochrane Database Syst Rev 2003;(3):CD002969.

84. Breitbart W: Spirituality and meaning in supportive care: spirituality- and meaning-centered group psychotherapy interventions in advanced cancer. *Support Care Cancer.* 2002; 10(4):272–280.

85. Cassell ES: The nature of suffering and the goals of medicine. *N Engl J Med.* 1982;306.639–645.

86. Daaleman TP, VandeCreek L: Placing religion and spirituality in end-of-life care. *JAMA.* 2000;284(19):2514–2517.

87. Kagawa-Singer M, Blackhall LJ: Negotiating cross-cultural issues at the end of life: "You got to go where he lives." *JAMA.* 2001;286(23):2993–3001.

88. Lo B, Ruston D, Kates LW, Arnold RM, Cohen CB, Faber-Langendoen K, Pantilat SZ, Puchalski CM, Quill TR, Rabow MW, Schreiber S, Sulmasy DP, Tulsky JA for the Working Group on Religious and Spiritual Issues at the End of Life: Discussing religious and spiritual issues at the end of life: a practical guide for physicians. *JAMA.* 2002;287:749–754.

89. Neuberger J: *Caring for Dying People of Different Faiths.* Baltimore: Mosby, 1994.

90. Post SG, Puchalski CM, Larson DB: Physicians and patient spirituality: professional boundaries, competency, and ethics. *Ann Intern Med.* 2000;132:578–583.

91. Sloan RP, Bagiella E, VandeCreek L, Hover M, Casalone C, Jinpu Hirsch T, Hasan Y, Kreger R, Poulos P: Should physicians prescribe religious activities? *N Engl J Med.* 2000; 342(25):1913–1916.

92. Sulmasy DP: Is medicine a spiritual practice? *Acad Med.* 1999;74(9):1002–1005.

93. Christakis MA, Sachs GA: The role of prognosis in clinical decision making. *J Gen Intern Med.* 1996;11(7):422–425.

94. Ersek M, Kagawa-Singer M, Barnes D, Blackhall L, Koenig BA: Multicultural considerations in the use of advance directives. *Oncol Nurs Forum.* 1998;25(10):1683–1690.

95. Hallenbeck J, Goldstein MK: Decisions at the end-of-life: cultural considerations beyond medical ethics. *Generations.* 1999;23(1):4–29.

96. Hern HE Jr, Koenig BA, Moore LJ, Marshall PA: The difference that culture can make in end-of-life decisionmaking. *Camb Q Healthc Ethics.* 1998;7(1):27–40.

97. Hopp FP, Duffy SA: Racial variations in end-of-life care. *J Am Geriatr Soc.* 2000;48(6):658–63.

98. Kolarik RC, Arnold RM, Fischer GS, Tulsky JA: Objectives for advance care planning. *J Palliat Med.* 2002;5(5):697–704.

99. Krakauer EL, Crenner C, Fox K: Barriers to optimum end-of-life care for minority patients. *J Am Geriatr Soc.* 2002;50(1): 182–190.

100. Teno JM, Clarridge BR, Casey V, Welch LC, Wetle T, Shield R, Mor V: Family perspectives on end-of-life care at the last place of care. *JAMA.* 2004;291(1):88–93.

101. Teno JM, Stevens M, Spernak S, Lynn J: Role of written advance directives in decision making: insights from qualitative and quantitative data. *J Gen Intern Med.* 1998;13(7):439–446.

102. Brody H, Campbell ML, Faber-Langendoen K, Ogle KS: Withdrawing intensive life-sustaining treatment—recommendations for compassionate clinical management. *N Engl J Med.* 1997; 336(9):652–657.

103. Ellershaw J, Ward C: Care of the dying patient: the last hours or days of life. *BMJ.* 2003;32:30–34.

104. Krakauer EL, Penson RT, Truog RD, King LA, Chabner BA, Lynch TJ Jr: Sedation for intractable distress of a dying patient: acute palliative care and the principle of double effect. *Oncologist.* 2000;5(1):53–62.

105. Pickett M, Yancey D: Symptoms of the dying. In: McCorkle R, Grant R, Frank-Stromborg M, Baird S, (eds): *Cancer Nursing: A Comprehensive Textbook,* 2nd ed. Philadelphia: W.B. Saunders, 1998:1157–1182.

106. Rousseau P: Management of symptoms in the actively dying patient. In: Berger AM, Portenoy RK, Weissman DE, (eds): *Principles & Practice of Palliative Care & Supportive Oncology,* 2nd ed. Philadelphia: Lippincott Williams & Wilkins, 2002: 789–798.

107. Ventafridda V, Ripamonti C, De Conno F, Tamburini M, Cassileth BR: Symptom prevalence and control during cancer patients' last days of life. *J Palliat Care*. 1990;6(3):7–11.

108. American College of Physicians—American Society of Internal Medicine End-of-Life Care Consensus Panel: Ethics manual. 4th ed. *Ann Intern Med*. 1998;128(7):576–594.

109. Council on Ethical and Judicial Affairs, American Medical Association: Medical futility in end-of-life care. *JAMA*. 1999; 281(10):937–941.

110. Berry P, Griffie J: Planning for the actual death. In: Ferrell BR, Coyle N (eds): *Textbook of Palliative Nursing*. New York: Oxford University Press, 2001:382–394.

111. Block SD, Billings JA: Patient requests to hasten death. Evaluation and management in terminal care. *Arch Intern Med*. 1994;154:2039–2047.

112. Campbell ML, Guzman JA: Impact of a proactive approach to improve end-of-life care in a medical ICU. *Chest*. 2003;123(1): 266–271.

113. Cherny NI, Portenoy RK: Sedation in the management of refractory symptoms: guidelines for evaluation and treatment. *J Palliat Care*. 1994;10(2):31–38.

114. Council on Ethical and Judicial Affairs, American Medical Association: Decisions near the end of life. *JAMA*. 1992;267: 2229–2233.

115. Ganzini L, Volicer L, Nelson W, Derse A: Pitfalls in assessment of decision-making capacity. *Psychosomatics*. 2003;44(3): 237–243.

116. Joranson DE, Gilson AM: Legal and regulatory issues in the management of pain. In: Graham AW, Schultz TK, et al., (eds): Principles of Addiction Medicine, 3rd ed. Chevy Chase, MD: American Society of Addiction Medicine, 2003:1465–1474.

117. Pain and Policy Studies Group: Achieving Balance in Federal and State Pain Policy: a Guide to Evaluation, 2nd ed. Madison, Wisconsin: University of Wisconsin Comprehensive Cancer Center, 2003. Available at www.medsch.wisc.edu/painpolicy/2003_balance/.

118. Koenig BA: Cultural diversity in decision-making about care at the end-of-life. In: Cassel CK, Field MJ, (eds): *Approaching*

Death: Improving Care at the End of Life. Washington, D.C.: Institute of Medicine, National Academy Press, 1997:363–382.

119. Meisel A, Snyder L, Quill T for the American College of Physicians—American Society of Internal Medicine End-of-Life Care Consensus Panel: Seven legal barriers to end-of-life care: myths, realities, and grains of truth. *JAMA.* 2000; 284(19):2495–2501.

120. Prendergast TJ, Luce JM: Increasing incidence of withholding and withdrawal of life support from the critically ill. *Am J Respir Crit Care Med.* 1997;155(1):15–20.

121 Quill TE, Cassel CK: Nonabandonment: a central obligation for physicians. *Ann Intern Med.* 1995;122(5):368–374.

122. Quill TE, Lo B, Brock DW: Palliative options of last resort: a comparison of voluntarily stopping eating and drinking, terminal sedation, physician-assisted suicide, and voluntary active euthanasia. *JAMA.* 1997;278(23):2099–2104.

123. Truog RD, Cist AF, Brackett SE, Burns JP, Curley MA, Danis M, DeVita MA, Rosenbaum SH, Rothenberg DM, Sprung CL, Webb SA, Wlody GS, Hurford WE: Recommendations for end-of-life care in the intensive care unit: The Ethics Committee of the Society of Critical Care Medicine. *Crit Care Med.* 2001;29(12):2332–2348.

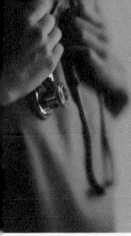

AMERICAN NURSES ASSOCIATION POSITION STATEMENT ON PAIN MANAGEMENT AND CONTROL OF DISTRESSING SYMPTOMS IN DYING PATIENTS

SUMMARY

In the context of the caring relationship (American Nurses Association, 2003), nurses perform a primary role in the assessment and management of pain and other distressing symptoms in dying patients. Therefore, nurses must use effective doses of medications prescribed for symptom control and nurses have a moral obligation to advocate on behalf of the patient when prescribed medication is insufficiently managing pain and other distressing symptoms. The increasing titration of medication to achieve adequate symptom control is ethically justified.

BACKGROUND

Nursing is the prevention of illness, the alleviation of suffering, and the protection, promotion, and restoration of health in the care of individuals, families, groups, communities, and populations (American Nurses Association, 2003). When the restoration of health is no longer possible, the focus of nursing care is

ANA Position Statement on Pain Management and Care of Distressing Symptoms in Dying Patients (Reprinted with permission from American Nurses Association, ANA Position Statement on Pain Management and Control of Distressing Symptoms in Dying Patients, ©2003 Nursesbooks.org, Silver Spring, MD.

assuring a comfortable, dignified death and the highest possible quality of remaining life. One of the major concerns of dying patients and their families is the fear of intractable pain during the dying process. Overwhelming pain and other distressing symptoms are related to sleeplessness, loss of morale, fatigue, irritability, restlessness, withdrawal, and other serious problems for the dying patient (Schickedanz, 2001; Ferrell & Coyle, 2001). Nurses are essential to the assessment and management of pain and other distressing symptoms as they generally have the most frequent and continuous patient contact. In planning nursing care, patients have the right to appropriate assessment and management of pain and other distressing symptoms. Pain and symptom management must be respected and supported (JCAHO, 2003).

The assessment and management of pain and other distressing symptoms must be based on an informed understanding of the individual patient's values and goals and his/her emotional, physical and spiritual needs as well as on an understanding of the pathophysiology of the disease state and evidence based palliative care practice. (Pierce, Dalton, & Duffey, 2001); National Pharmaceutical Council, 2001). One goal of nursing interventions for dying patients is to maximize comfort. When pain and other distressing symptoms are present, the patient should have appropriate and sufficient medication by appropriate routes to control symptoms, in whatever dosage, and by whatever route is needed to control symptoms as perceived by the patient. (American Nurses Association, 2001:§1; Pasero & McCaffrey, 2001) The nurse-patient relationship is a significant moral relationship, as such nurses must advocate on behalf of patients to ensure effective symptom control at the end of life.

REFERENCES

American Nurses Association (2003). Nursing's Social Policy Statement. Washington, DC: Nursesbooks.org

American Nurses Association (2001). Code of Ethics for Nurses With Interpretive Statements. Provision 1. Washington, DC: American Nurses Publishing

Ferrell, B.R., & Coyle, N. (2001). Palliative Nursing. New York: Oxford Press.

Joint Commission on Accreditation of Healthcare Organizations (JCAHO, 2003). Patient Rights and Organization Ethics Standard RI.1.2.9. Washington, DC: JCAHO

National Pharmaceutical Council. (2001). Pain: Current Understanding of Assessment Management and Treatments. December. P. 21

Pasero, C. & McCaffrey, M. (2001). Appropriate pain control. American Journal of Nursing 101 (11):13. December 2002

Pierce, S.F., Dalton, J.A. & Duffey, M. (2001). The nurse's ethical obligation to relieve pain: Actualizing the moral mandate. Journal of Nursing Law 7(4):19–29.

Schickedanz, L. (2001). Nursing Principles of Pain Management. p. 1

Effective Date:	December 5, 2003
Status:	Revised Position Statement
Originated by:	Center for Ethics & Human Rights Advisory Board
Adopted by:	ANA Board of Directors

RELATED PAST ACTION

1. Code for Nurses with Interpretive Statements, 1985.
2. Position Statement on Nurses' Participation in Capital Punishment, 1988.

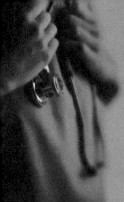

Appendix D

HPNA POSITION STATEMENT ON VALUE OF PROFESSIONAL NURSE IN END-OF-LIFE CARE

BACKGROUND

Nurses spend more time with patients and their families who are facing the end of life than any other member of the health-care team.[1] As members of the largest healthcare profession, nurses have long advocated for attention to quality of life. Achieving quality of life, especially at the end of life, is contingent upon competent, 'state of the art' professional nursing care. Nursing pioneers in palliative care, Florence Wald, Cicely Saunders (also a physician), and Jeanne Quint Benoliel, have emphasized that those in need of care at the end of life merit "the most competent, expert, evidence-based care provided in a way that embodies compassion, respect for dignity, and an appreciation for the whole person and the family."[2p. xiii–xv] In 1962, registered nurse Harriet Goetz published an approach to care for the dying that focused on open communication with the patient and family and symptom management techniques such as atropine for secretions and environmental adjustments (such as making the room pleasant, soft lighting, and so on), to provide comfort.[3] The work of these nurse leaders forged the way towards the current standard practice for comprehensive and compassionate care at the end of life.

HPNA Position Statement on Value of Professional Nurse in End-of-Life Care. Reproduced, with permission, from the Hospice and Palliative Nurses Association, Pittsburgh, PA. www.hpna.org.

Competency based nursing practice at the end of life includes expert assessment skills, critical thinking, comprehensive pain, and symptom management, and the acquisition of knowledge, attitudes and skills in areas related to the phases of wellness and illness at the end of life. Ferrell emphasized that the management of a "single physical symptom, such as dyspnea, requires expert knowledge of physiology, numerous pharmacological treatments, nondrug interventions and psychological support to ease the distress of patient and family experiencing this symptom."[2p. xiii–xv] End-stage illness usually presents with not only one, but multiple and often complex symptoms that affect the body, mind, and spirit in tangential means, driving the professional nurse to employ highly trained skills and provide holistic care that is consistent with the goals of the patient and family. Individualized professional nursing care at this time of life has never been so critical to maximize autonomy, dignity, healing, and comfort.

When faced with a serious illness, people turn to their nurse or nurse practitioner for education, support, and guidance. Nurses are intimately involved in all aspects of end-of-life care. Professional nurses face end-of-life situations whether they work in hospitals, homes, long-term care facilities, clinics, universities and schools, industry, or prisons. They are the primary team members who coordinate, assess, direct, and evaluate patient care needs that arise during the illness experience. With their knowledge about the physical, psychosocial, and spiritual dimensions of life-limiting and terminal illness, nurses are central in assuring the comfort, autonomy, and healing of patients and families.

The professional nurse is also a key player in moving the healthcare team towards a recognition of end-of-life care situations and the comfort care and psychological support that are required.[4] Professional nursing at the end of life is grounded in keeping the positive traditions of past practices while shaping care for the future that will meet the evolving needs of the sick and dying. The professional nurse establishes and supports the methods and means to assure these outcomes are met.

POSITION STATEMENT

It is the position of HPNA Board of Directors that professional nursing care is critical to achieving the patients', families', and communities' goals of care at the end of life. Support of hospice and palliative care research and education is necessary to ensure that care is evidence-based, effective, and appropriate.

DEFINITION OF TERMS

Critical thinking—process of utilizing cognitive skills to analyze, apply standards, discriminate, seek information/data, reason logically, predict and transform knowledge. Critical thinkers exhibit habits of the mind: confidence, contextual perspective, creativity, flexibility, inquisitiveness, intellectual integrity, intuition, open-mindedness, perseverance, and reflection.[5]

End-of-Life Care—nursing care for people who are experiencing life-limiting progressive illness(es).[6]

Evidence-based practice—practice that is based on research, clinical expertise, and patient preferences that guide decisions about the healthcare of individual patients. Evidence-based nursing de-emphasizes ritual, isolated, and unsystematic clinical experience, ungrounded opinions, and traditions as a basis for nursing practice. It stresses the use of research findings, quality improvement data (as appropriate), other operational and evaluation data, the consensus of recognized experts, and affirmed experience to substantiate practice.[7]

REFERENCES

1. Ferrell BR, Grant M, Virani R. Strengthening nursing education to improve end-of-life care. *Nursing Outlook.* 1999;47:252–256

2. Ferrell BR. Forward. In: Matzo M, Sherman D, eds. *Palliative Care Nursing: Quality care to the end of life.* New York, NY: Springer Publishing Company; 2001:xiii–xv.

3. Poleto M. Hospice care: Underutilized and misunderstood. In: Dochterman J, Grace HY, eds. *Current Issues in Nursing.* St. Louis, MO: Mosby; 2001:175–181.

4. Zinc M, Titus L. Ethical issues and resource for nurses across the continuum. In: Dochterman J, Grace HY, eds. *Current Issues in Nursing.* St. Louis, MO: Mosby; 2001:568–575.
5. Rubenfeld M, Scheffer B. Critical thinking: What is it and how do we teach it? In: Dochterman J, Grace HY, eds. *Current Issues in Nursing.* St. Louis, MO: Mosby; 2001:125–132.
6. Hospice and Palliative Nurses Association. *Definition of End of Life Care.* Pittsburgh, PA: HPNA; 2003.
7. Goode C, Krugman M. Evidenced-based practice: A tool for clinical and managerial decision making. In: Dochterman J, Grace HY, eds. *Current Issues in Nursing.* St. Louis, MO: Mosby; 2001:60–68.

Approved by the HPNA Board of Directors October 2003

To obtain copies of HPNA Position Statements, contact the National Office at
Penn Center West One, Suite 229, Pittsburgh, PA 15276
Phone (412) 787-9301
Fax (412) 787-9305
Website www.HPNA.org

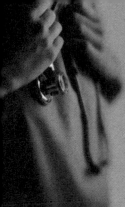

HPNA POSITION STATEMENT ON PROVIDING OPIOIDS AT THE END OF LIFE

BACKGROUND

Pain management is integral to quality hospice and palliative care.[1,2] Experts advocate for adequate analgesia to be provided to all patients in pain, including older adults, infants and children, non-verbal patients, non-English-speaking people and those with active or a history of substance abuse.[1–6] Providing effective pain management should be a primary objective in every clinical setting—especially those settings that provide care to dying patients.

Although there is agreement that the goals of palliative care must focus on the prevention and relief of pain and suffering, clinicians, patients, and families may be reluctant to use opioids to achieve this goal in patients who are dying.[7,8] This hesitancy may stem from the fear that administering opioids depresses respirations, thereby hastening death. However, there is no convincing scientific evidence that administering opioids, even in very high doses, accelerates death.[9–13] In fact, numerous clinical studies demonstrate no significant association among opioid use, respiratory depression, and shortened survival.[10,12,14–20] Respiratory depression and other changes in breathing are part of the dying process and are more likely to be from disease and multi-system organ failure than from opioids.[16,21]

Despite the lack of evidence that opioids hasten death, some clinicians continue to believe that administering opioids can accelerate the dying process; for this reason, they seek moral justification for providing aggressive pain management. The rule of double effect[22] provides ethical justification for the use of opioids in dying patients even if there is a risk of hastening death. According to the rule of double effect, four conditions must be satisfied to establish a clinician's act as morally permissible:

- The act must be good or morally neutral, regardless of its consequences; relief of pain and suffering by administering opioids is a priority in hospice and palliative care and therefore is a "good act."

- The clinician must intend the good effect (relief of the patient's pain and suffering); although the bad effect (i.e., death) may be foreseen and permitted, it is not the clinician's intended effect.

- The bad effect must not be the means by which the good effect is achieved; in other words, the patient does not need to die in order to be relieved of pain.

- The benefits of the good effect must outweigh the burdens of the bad effect; in this case, the benefits of achieving pain relief outweigh the minimal risk of hastening death.[23]

Professional organizations, state lawmakers, and the U.S. Supreme Court have asserted their support for administering opioids at the end of life by explicitly or implicitly invoking the rule of double effect.[2,24–26] Thus, fear of hastening death as a result of opioid administration does not justify the withholding of pain medication. In contrast, assisted suicide and euthanasia are not generally seen as moral acts under the rule of double effect because the primary, explicit intent in these cases is to cause death. The difference between these acts (i.e., assisted suicide and euthanasia) and administering opioids for pain relief is that causing death, even for the relief of suffering, is usually not seen as a good or a morally neutral act.[27]

There is broad consensus among professional groups, ethicists, courts, and many state legislatures that clinicians have a duty to administer opioids for pain relief to patients at the end of life.[2, 26, 28] Education and support are necessary to ensure that clinicians in all settings understand their obligation to relieve pain and suffering and to achieve skill and comfort in the clinical activities that are necessary to meet this goal.[2,29–31]

POSITION STATEMENT

The Hospice and Palliative Nurses Association (HPNA) is committed to compassionate care of persons at the end of life. It is the position of the HPNA Board of Directors that:

- Hospice and palliative care nurses and organizations must affirm that pain management should continue throughout the dying process
- Hospice and palliative care nurses and organizations must affirm that comprehensive pain management is a hallmark of excellent hospice and palliative care
- Hospice and palliative care nurses and organizations must affirm that patients in all clinical settings have the right to receive adequate pain relief throughout their illness experience
- Hospice and palliative care nurses and organizations must recognize that the administration of opioids to alleviate pain at the end of life is consistent with widely accepted ethical and legal principles
- Hospice and palliative care nurses and organizations must recognize that administering opioids to relieve pain in dying patients is ethically and legally different from assisted suicide and euthanasia; the intent of the former is to relieve pain, while the intent of assisted suicide and euthanasia is to cause death as a means of alleviating suffering
- Hospice and palliative care nurses and organizations must advocate for education across health care settings to enable clinicians in recognizing their responsibility to relieve pain at the end of life. This education should include information about the lack of empirical evidence that opioids shorten life as well as the ethical and legal acceptability of administering opioids in doses sufficient to relieve pain.

- Health care professionals and organizations must support nurses and other clinicians in discerning between ethically justifiable, legally permitted palliative care interventions and those interventions which may not be ethically justifiable and/or legally permitted
- Health care organizations should develop policies regarding the administration of opioids for pain relief.
- Hospice and palliative care nurses must recognize that the risk of hastening death by administering opioids to patients with life-limiting, progressive illnesses is minimal, particularly when administration occurs by or under the supervision of clinicians skilled in pain and symptom management and is consistent with established pain management guidelines.
- Clinicians across clinical settings must reflect on their responsibility to alleviate pain and suffering. This reflection must include careful deliberation regarding standards of practice and the array of interventions that are essential to meeting the goals of palliative care.
- Clinicians who regularly care for dying patients must achieve comfort and skill in providing aggressive pain management.

DEFINITION OF TERMS

Assisted Suicide: Making a means of suicide (for example, providing lethal doses of medications) available to a patient with knowledge of the patient's intention to kill him- or herself.[22]

Euthanasia: An act that is performed by a clinician with the intent to end the patient's life (for example, administering a lethal injection); also called "mercy killing."[32]

Rule of Double Effect: A bioethical concept that provides moral justification for an action that has two foreseen effects: one good and one bad. The key factor is the intent of the person performing the act. If the intent is good (e.g., relief of pain and suffering) then the act is morally justifiable even if it causes a foreseeable but unintended result (e.g., hastening of death).[22,23,25] Also referred to as the "doctrine of double effect."

REFERENCES

1. Hospice and Palliative Nurses Association. Position statement on pain. Available at: http://www.hpna.org/positions.asp. Accessed October 31, 2003.

2. American Nurses Association. Position Statement: Promotion of comfort and relief of pain in dying patients. Available at: www.nursingworld.org/readroom/position/ethics/etpain.htm. Accessed October 31, 2003.

3. American Geriatrics Society. The management of persistent pain in older persons. *J Am Geriatr Soc.* 2002;50(6 Suppl): S205–224.

4. American Society of Pain Management Nurses. ASPMN position statement: Pain management in patients with addictive disease. Available at: http://www.aspmn.org/html/PSaddiction. htm. Accessed November 17, 2003.

5. McGrath P, Finley G. Pediatric pain: biological and social context. Seattle, WA: IASP Press; 2003.

6. McCaffery M, Pasero C. Pain. Clinical manual. 2nd ed. St. Louis: Mosby; 1999.

7. Solomon MZ, O'Donnell L, Jennings B, Guilfoy, V, Wolf, SM, Nolan, K, Jackson, R, Koch-Weser, D, Donnelley, S. Decisions near the end of life: professional views on life-sustaining treatments. *Amer J Pub Health.* 1993;83:14–23.

8. Volker DL. Oncology nurses' experiences with requests for assisted dying from terminally ill patients with cancer. *Oncology Nursing Forum.* 2001;28:39–49.

9. Fohr S. The double effect of pain medication: Separating myth from reality. *J Palliat Med.* 1998;1:315–328.

10. Campbell ML, Bizek KS, Thill M. Patient responses during rapid terminal weaning from mechanical ventilation: a prospective study. *Crit Care Med.* 1999;27:73–77.

11. Wall PD. The generation of yet another myth on the use of narcotics. *Pain.* 1997;73:121–122.

12. Wilson WC, Smedira NG, Fink C, McDowell JA, Luce JM. Ordering and administration of sedatives and analgesics during the withholding and withdrawal of life support from critically ill patients. *JAMA.* 1992;267:949–953.

13. Sykes N, Thorns A. The use of opioids and sedatives at the end of life. *Lancet Oncol.* 2003;4:312–318.

14. Walsh TD. Opiates and respiratory function in advanced cancer. *Recent Results Cancer Res.* 1984;89:115–117.

15. Citron ML, Johnston-Early A, Fossieck BE, Krasnow, SH, Franklin, R, Spagnolo, SV, Cohen, MH. Safety and efficacy of continuous intravenous morphine for severe cancer pain. *Am J Med.* 1984;77:199–204.

16. Grond S, Zech D, Schug SA, Lynch J, Lehmann KA. Validation of World Health Organization guidelines for cancer pain relief during the last days and hours of life. *J Pain Symptom Manage.* 1991;6:411–422.

17. Walsh T, Rivera N, Kaiko R. Oral morphine and respiratory function amongst hospice inpatients with advanced cancer. *Support Care Ca.* 2003;11:780–784.

18. Morita T, Ichiki T, Tsunoda J, Inoue S, Chihara S. A prospective study on the dying process in terminally ill cancer patients. *Am J Hospice Palliat Care.* 1998;15:217–222.

19. Morita T, Tsunoda J, Inoue S, Chihara S. Effects of high dose opioids and sedatives on survival in terminally ill cancer patients. *J Pain Symptom Manage.* 2001;21:282–289.

20. Bercovitch M, Waller A, Adunsky A. High dose morphine use in the hospice setting. A database survey of patient characteristics and effect on life expectancy. *Cancer.* 1999;86:871–877.

21. Buchan ML, Tolle SW. Pain relief for dying persons: dealing with physicians' fears and concerns. *J Clinic Ethics.* 1995;6: 53–61.

22. American Nurses Association. Position Statement: Assisted Suicide. December 8, 1994. Available at: http://www.ana.org/readroom/position/ethics/etsuic.htm. Accessed May 5, 2003.

23. Beauchamp TL, Childress JF. Principles of biomedical ethics. 5th ed. New York: Oxford University Press; 2001.

24. American Academy of Hospice and Palliative Medicine. Position Statement: Comprehensive end-of-life care and physician-assisted suicide. *AAHPM* [website]. Available at:http://www.aahpm.org/positions/suicide.html. Accessed November 5, 2003.

25. American Nurses Association. Code of ethics for nurses with interpretive statements. Washington, DC: American Nurses Association; 2001.
26. Natural Death Act. *Revised Code of Washington*. Vol RCW 70.122.010; 1992.
27. Sulmasy DP, Pellegrino ED. The rule of double effect: clearing up the double talk. *Arch of Inter Med.* 1999;159(6):545–550.
28. Haddad A. Ethics in action. Your cancer patient's pain. RN. 1997;60(11):21–22.
29. Pellegrino ED. Emerging ethical issues in palliative care. *JAMA.* 1998;279(19):1521–1522.
30. Pierce SF, Dalton JA, Duffey M. The nurse's ethical obligation to relieve pain: actualizing the moral mandate. *J Nurs Law.* 2001; 7(4):19–29.
31. Kennedy-Schwarz J. Pain management. A moral imperative. *Am J Nurs.* 2000;100(8):49–50.
32. American Nurses A. Position Statement: Active Euthanasia. *American Nurses Association, Task Force on the Nurses' Role in End-of-Life Decisions, Center for Ethics and Human Rights* [Website]. December 8, 1994. Available at: http://www.ana.org/readroom/position/ethics/ctcuth.htm. Accessed 03-04, 2000.

Related HPNA Position Statements: Pain, approved October 2003

Approved by the HPNA Board of Directors April 2004

To obtain copies of HPNA Position Statements, contact the National Office at
Penn Center West One, Suite 229, Pittsburgh, PA 15276
Phone (412) 787-9301
Fax (412) 787-9305
Website: www.HPNA.org

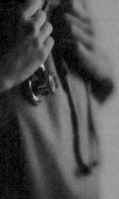

HPNA POSITION STATEMENT ON ARTIFICIAL NUTRITION AND HYDRATION IN END-OF-LIFE CARE

BACKGROUND

Patients with life-limiting, progressive illness often experience a decline in appetite, loss of interest in eating and drinking, and weight loss. Some patients may experience dysphagia, which also decreases oral intake. At some point in the illness trajectory, most patients will either be unable to take food and fluids by mouth or will refuse food, including their favorite foods.[1,2] These changes can cause distress, especially for families and other caregivers, and raise questions about artificial nutrition and hydration (ANH).[2]

The decision to implement ANH should consider probable benefits and burdens of the therapy. Artificial nutrition and hydration has traditionally been used to meet several therapeutic goals: 1) prolong life; 2) prevent aspiration pneumonia; 3) maintain independence and physical function; and 4) decrease suffering and discomfort at the end of life.[3] There are few well-designed studies, however, that have examined whether or not ANH is effective in meeting these goals. The empirical evidence that has been published indicates that ANH often does not affect these clinical objectives. For example, studies show that tube feeding does not appear to prolong life in most patients with

HPNA Position Statement on Artificial Nutrition and Hydration in End-of-Life Care. Reproduced, with permission, from the Hospice and Palliative Nurses Association, Pittsburgh, PA. www.hpna.org.

life-limiting, progressive diseases; moreover, complications from tube placement may increase mortality.[4–6] Furthermore, artificially-delivered nutrition does not protect against aspiration and in some patient populations may actually *increase* the risk of aspiration and its complications.[3,4,7–9] Finally, research has shown that artificial nutrition and nutritional supplements do not enhance frail elders' strength and physical function.[4,10,11]

One of the most important aims of hospice and palliative care is to minimize suffering and discomfort. Many patients, families, and other caregivers fear that undernourished patients may experience hunger. They may also believe that dehydration results in troublesome symptoms such as thirst, dry mouth, headache, delirium, nausea, vomiting, and abdominal cramps.[12] Contrary to expectations, however, studies show that most actively dying patients do not experience hunger even if they have inadequate caloric intake.[13] Many patients may experience thirst, but this symptom is not associated with fluid status; therefore, parenteral fluids are unlikely to alleviate thirst.[12] Headache, nausea and vomiting and abdominal cramps are not associated with dehydration in terminally-ill patients.[14] Dry mouth is common, but is not improved by tube feeding or intravenous hydration; conscientious mouth care and small amounts of fluid and ice chips effectively relieve dry mouth.[13–15]

In addition to lack of evidence for the beneficial effects of ANH on patient comfort, the possible complications of therapy discourage its use in most patients at the end of life. Parenteral fluids and total parenteral nutrition can cause considerable discomfort with repeated venipunctures and iatrogenic infections. Fluid therapy has also been reported to worsen edema and increase respiratory tract secretions, although these outcomes are not strongly supported by research.[14] Tube feedings are associated with increased infection, fluid overload and skin excoriation around the tube.[4] Since many tube-fed patients are not offered food, even if they are able to eat, they may be deprived of human contact and the pleasure of eating.[15,16] Other discomforts associated with tube feedings include exacerbation of nausea, vomiting, and diarrhea, as well as throat and nose pain from nasogastric tubes. Finally, therapies such as ANH that require the use of tubes increase the likelihood that patients will be restrained.[16–18] Physical restraints are distressing and often increase patient agitation.[19]

In addition to the evaluation of the clinical benefits and burdens of ANH, decision-making regarding the use of ANH must occur in the context of an open discussion and incorporate the patient's values and goals for care. When patients are incapable of understanding their prognosis and treatment choices or are unable to express their wishes, advance directives and surrogate decision makers must be consulted.

The right of competent adults to decide whether or not to accept or refuse specific medical therapies is now well established through legal precedent. Artificial nutrition and hydration is considered medical treatment and thus can be requested or refused.[1,20] This right reflects respect for patient autonomy.[21] Competent adults may express their decision about ANH and other therapies through advance directives, which should guide care planning at the end of life if the person is no longer able to make decisions or express his or her wishes. The right of parents to forego or withdraw ANH for children who are unlikely to benefit from the therapy also needs to be honored.[22]

Providing food and fluids is a fundamental caregiving activity. When caregivers witness gradual decline in the ability to take food and fluids, they may feel compelled to ensure that adequate nutrition and fluid are provided. They may fear that the patient will suffer as she or he "starves" to death or dies of dehydration.[2,16,23] Therefore, families and other caregivers need to be presented with accurate information about the burdens and benefits of ANH.

The provision of nutrition is also a significant opportunity for social interaction between caregiver and patient. Artificial nutrition and hydration denies caregivers this opportunity. Artificial nutrition and hydration may be used inappropriately in patients with conditions such as dysphagia that hinder oral intake. Many of these patients can continue to eat and drink, provided that adaptive feeding and hygiene techniques are utilized.[15,24] Speech therapists can be particularly helpful in identifying risk factors for complications of oral and tube feeding. They also can teach staff and family caregivers safe feeding techniques.

When feeding activities are no longer possible or reasonable, families and other caregivers should be educated and supported in other ways to provide comfort and social interaction. It is important that they understand that decreased oral intake is a natural, nonpainful part of the dying process.

Despite the evidence that ANH should not be routinely used for patients at the end of life, one should not categorically rule out its use in all patients. For example, some patients may benefit from fluid therapy, such as patients with opioid toxicity and delirium associated with dehydration.[25,26] Traditionally, hospice providers have been reluctant to provide ANH to patients and at times, this reluctance has translated into policies that deny ANH to all hospice patients. In contrast, acute care settings routinely provide aggressive fluid replacement and at times invasive nutritional therapies without regard to the lack of positive outcomes associated with the therapy.[25,26] Given the wide spectrum of patients now treated by hospice and palliative care teams, some experts suggest that a "middle road" between universal treatment and universal nontreatment fosters the most effective decision-making around ANH.[26,27] For example, policies and practices might discourage the use of ANH in situations where ANH is unlikely to benefit patients but allow a trial of ANH in situations where patients might benefit (e.g., using fluid therapy for delirium associated with dehydration).

In addition to medical indications for ANH, nurses should recognize specific religious and cultural groups for whom withholding or withdrawing ANH are considered immoral. Although members of these groups should not be stereotyped and assumptions about religious and cultural beliefs should be avoided, sociocultural and spiritual considerations need to be incorporated into decisions about initiating and withdrawing ANH.[28,29]

POSITION STATEMENT

The Hospice and Palliative Nurses Association (HPNA) is committed to compassionate care of persons at the end of life. The HPNA believes that the decision to initiate, withhold, or withdraw ANH should be made by the patient and family with accurate and nonjudgmental input from the healthcare team. Ideally, this decision is also documented in an advance directive and clearly communicated to the surrogate decision maker and healthcare team. It is the position of the HPNA Board of Directors to:

- Promote the education of healthcare providers to ensure that they understand the clinical, legal, and ethical issues regarding the use of ANH.

- Support education of patient, family and other caregivers about the dying process and its effects on nutrition and fluid status.

- Caregivers should be taught to enhance the patient's comfort by providing frequent oral and skin care, effective and timely symptom management, and psycho-spiritual support. Support caregivers in coping with feelings of helplessness, loss, and fear.

- Recognize that in specific situations, ANH may be clinically beneficial. ANH may also be initiated or continued to honor the beliefs and values of some cultural and religious groups.

- Encourage nurses to collaborate with speech therapists, nutritionists, and other healthcare providers to identify and implement strategies that enable caregivers to provide oral nutrition and fluids safely and effectively, as an alternative to ANH.

- Promote the use of a decision-making process that examines the benefits and burdens of ANH and includes the patient's clinical condition, goals, and values.

- Acknowledge and support the established, legal and moral right of competent patients to refuse unwanted treatment, including ANH.

- Acknowledge and support the family's or other surrogate's role as decision-maker in cases where a patient is unable to make his or her wishes known or is unable to evaluate the benefits and burdens of artificial nutrition or hydration.

- Promote the use of advance directives such as living wills or the legal assignment of durable power of attorney for health care to document choices and values that should guide care at the end of life in the event that decision-making capacity is lost.

- Promote early discussions about the goals of care and treatment choices, including the expected benefits and burdens of possible end-of-life interventions including ANH, prior to treatment initiation, refusal, or withdrawal.

- Encourage policies that guide a decision making process for resolving disagreements about care among patients, families, surrogates, and healthcare team members.

- Support research on the outcomes of ANH in diverse groups of hospice and palliative care patients.

DEFINITION OF TERMS

Advance Directives: documents that provide written instructions regarding healthcare choices when a person is no longer able to make or to communicate decisions. Two major types of advance directives are the: 1) *living will,* which gives instructions regarding specific medical procedures and therapies that should be provided or foregone in specific circumstances (e.g., in terminal illness, dementia, persistent vegetative state); and 2) *durable power of attorney for health care (DPOA-HC),* in which one person assigns another person the authority to make healthcare decisions on his/her behalf in the event that he or she becomes incompetent.[21] Advance directives provide a means by which autonomy is respected when the person is no longer competent. Laws regulating advance directives differ from state to state.

Artificial hydration: administration of fluid through non-oral means; routes include intravenous or subcutaneous (also called hypodermoclysis), rectal (proctoclysis), and enteral.[30]

Artificial nutrition: nonoral, mechanical feeding either by the intravenous or enteral route. Enteral feedings may be provided through either nasogastric tubes, or gastrostomy, esophagostomy, or jejunostomy tubes that are placed either endoscopically or in open surgical procedures. Intravenous nutrition is administered through a central line and often is called total parenteral nutrition(TPN).[15,30]

Autonomy: (From the Greek, *autos* "self"; *nomos* "rule" "government") a bioethical principle that is concerned with the ability and right of individuals to make decisions for themselves.[21] Autonomous decision makers are persons who can act: 1) intentionally; 2) with freedom from controlling influences and coercion; and 3) based on an understanding of the situation and choices.[21] Autonomy directs nurses and other healthcare providers to respect the choices of competent individuals regarding procedures and therapies.[31]

Competency: ability to perform a task;[21] in the context of end-of-life decision making, the term refers to the ability of patients to understand the diagnosis, prognosis and treatment choices, to make a reasoned judgment about different treatments, and to communicate their preferences for care. Competence often is differentiated from "capacity" in that the former indicates a legal judgment, decided in court, and the latter refers to a clinical judgment made by health professionals. In practice, however, there often is little practical difference between competence and capacity.[21]

Surrogate decision maker: a person authorized to make decisions on behalf of an incapacitated person; the authority is established through a legal document such as durable power of attorney for healthcare (DPOA-HC), a court proceeding, or as authorized by state laws.[21]

REFERENCES

1. Position statement on foregoing nutrition and fluid. *American Nurses Association.* Available at: http://www.nursingworld.org/readroom/position/ethics/etnutr.htm. Accessed February 4, 2003.
2. Twycross R, Lichter I. The terminal phase. In: Doyle D, Hanks G, MacDonald N, eds. *Oxford textbook of palliative medicine.* 2nd ed. New York: Oxford University Press; 1998:977–992.

3. Hallenbeck J. Fast facts and concepts #10: Tube feed or not tube feed? *J Palliat Med.* 2002;5(6):909–910.
4. Finucane TE, Christmas C, Travis K. Tube feeding in patients with advanced dementia: a review of the evidence. *JAMA.* 1999;282(14):1365–1370.
5. Mitchell SL, Kiely DK, Lipsitz LA. Does artificial enteral nutrition prolong the survival of institutionalized elders with chewing and swallowing problems? *J Gerontol A Biolog Sci Med Sci.* 1998;53(3):M207–213.
6. Rabeneck L, McCullough LB, Wray NP. Ethically justified, clinically comprehensive guidelines for percutaneous endoscopic gastrostomy tube placement. *Lancet.* 1997;349(9050): 496–498.
7. Cogen R, Weinryb J, Pomerantz C, Fenstemacher P. Complications of jejunostomy tube feeding in nursing facility patients. *Am J Gastroenterol.* 1991;86(11):1610–1613.
8. Finucane TE, Bynum JP. Use of tube feeding to prevent aspiration pneumonia. *Lancet.* 1996;348(9039):1421–1424.
9. Kadakia SC, Sullivan HO, Starnes E. Percutaneous endoscopic gastrostomy or jejunostomy and the incidence of aspiration in 79 patients. *Am J Surg.* 1992;164(2):114–118.
10. Fiatarone M, O'Neill E, Ryan N, et al. Exercise training and nutritional supplementation for physical frailty in very elderly people. *N Engl J Med.* 1994;330(25):1769–1775.
11. Kaw M, Sekas G. Long-term follow-up of consequences of percutaneous endoscopic gastrostomy (PEG) tubes in nursing home patients. *Dig Dis Sci.* 1994;39(4):738–743.
12. Ellershaw JE. Dehydration and the dying patient. *J Pain Symptous Manage.* 1995;10(3):192–197.
13. McCann RM, Hall WJ, Groth-Juncker A. Comfort care for terminally ill patients. The appropriate use of nutrition and hydration. *JAMA.* 1994;272(16):1263–1266.
14. Billings JA. Comfort measures for the terminally ill. Is dehydration painful? *J Am Geriatr Soc.* 1985;33(11):808–810.
15. Dahlin C, Goldsmith T. Dysphagia, dry mouth, and hiccups. In: Ferrell B, Coyle N, eds. *Textbook of Palliative Nursing.* New York: Oxford University Press; 2001:122–138.

16. Gillick MR. Rethinking the role of tube feeding in patients with advanced dementia. *N Engl J Med.* 2000; 342(3):206–210.

17. Quill TE. Utilization of nasogastric feeding tubes in a group of chronically ill, elderly patients in a community hospital. *Arch Intern Med.* 1989; 149(9):1937–1941.

18. Sullivan-Marx EM, Strumpf NE, Evans LK, Baumgarten M, Maislin G. Predictors of continued physical restraint use in nursing home residents following restraint reduction efforts. *J Am Geriatr Soc.* 1999;47(3):342–348.

19. Evans LK, Strumpf NE. Tying down the elderly. A review of the literature on physical restraint. *J Am Geriatr Soc.* 1989;37(1): 65–74.

20. Gostin LO. Deciding life and death in the courtroom. From Quinlan to Cruzan, Glucksberg, and Vacco—a brief history and analysis of constitutional protection of the 'right to die'. *JAMA.* 1997;278(18):1523–1528.

21. Beauchamp T, Childress J. *Principles of biomedical ethics.* 5th ed. New York: Oxford University Press; 2001.

22. Nelson LJ, Rushton CH, Cranford RE, Nelson RM, Glover JJ, Truog RD. Forgoing medically provided nutrition and hydration in pediatric patients. *J Law Med Ethics.* 1995;23(1):33–46.

23. Callahan CM, Haag KM, Buchanan NN, Nisi R. Decision-making for percutaneous endoscopic gastrostomy among older adults in a community setting. *J Am Geriatr Soc.* 1999;47(9): 1105–1109.

24. Langmore SE, Terpenning MS, Schork A, et al. Predictors of aspiration pneumonia: how important is dysphagia? *Dysphagia.* 1998;13(2):69–81.

25. Fainsinger RL, Bruera E. When to treat dehydration in a terminally ill patient? *Support Care Cancer.* 1997;5(3):205–211.

26. Choi YS, Billings JA. Changing perspectives on palliative care. *Oncology (Huntingt).* 2002;16(4):515–522.

27. Bruera E. The Choi and Billings article reviewed. *Oncology (Huntingt).* 2002;19(4):522–523.

28. Schostak RZ. Jewish ethical guidelines for resuscitation and artificial nutrition and hydration of the dying elderly. *J Med Ethics.* 1994;20(2):93–100.

29. Hamel R, DuBose ER. Views of the major faith traditions. In: Hamel R, ed. *Choosing death: Active euthanasia, religion, and the public debate.* Deerfield, IL: Trinity Press International; 1991: 45–77.

30. Kedziera P. Hydration, thirst, and nutrition. In: Ferrell B, Coyle N, eds. *Textbook of palliative nursing.* New York: Oxford University Press; 2001:156–163.

31. Daly BJ. Special challenges of withholding artificial nutrition and hydration. *J Gerontol Nurs.* 2000;26(9):25–31.

Approved by the HPNA Board of Directors June 2003

To obtain copies of HPNA Position Statements, contact the National Office at
Penn Center West One, Suite 229, Pittsburgh, PA 15276
Phone (412) 787-9301
Fax (412) 787-9305
Website www.HPNA.org

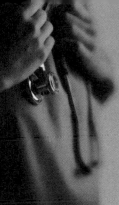

BACKGROUND

Studies have shown that use of complementary and alternative therapies in the United States is common and has increased over the past decade.[1] Reasons for this trend are varied, but include:

- Consumer dissatisfaction with conventional medical care and client-provider relationships;
- Increased consumer desire to participate in healthcare decision-making and in self-care;
- Consumer concerns regarding side effects of medications commonly used to control disease and symptoms;
- Growing numbers of people with chronic, incurable conditions;
- Concern about costs of healthcare; and
- Increasing cultural diversity of the American population and exposure to different models of health beliefs and healing.

Complementary therapies, also known as integrative therapies, encompass a broad spectrum of approaches and philosophies. Although many definitions exist, the National Center for Complementary and Alternative Medicine (NCCAM) describes

---

complementary and alternative medicine as "a group of diverse medical and health care systems, practices, and products that are not presently considered to be part of conventional medicine."[2] Another panel convened by the National Institutes of Health (NIH) defined complementary and alternative (CAM) therapies as:

> A broad domain of healing resources that encompasses all health systems, modalities, and practices and their accompanying theories and beliefs, other than those intrinsic to the politically dominant health system of a particular society or culture in a given historical period. CAM includes all such practices and ideas self-defined by their users as preventing or treating illness or promoting health and well-being. Boundaries within CAM and between the CAM domain and the domain of the dominant health system are not always sharp and fixed.[3]

Some authors use the terms "complementary" and "alternative" interchangeably; however, the latter term generally is reserved for those treatment approaches that are used *alone*. In contrast, complementary therapies are used *in addition to* conventional therapies.

The NCCAM categorizes complementary therapies into five domains: alternative medical systems, mind-body interventions, biologically-based therapies, manipulative and body-based methods, and energy therapies (see Table 1).[2] Over 200 complementary therapies have been identified. These therapies can involve interaction with providers (e.g., massage therapists, chiropractors) or unsupervised use (e.g., self-care). Self-use remains the predominant method of utilization.[1]

In general, complementary therapies are less well studied than conventional therapies. However, substantial scientific evidence exists for some complementary therapies. These approaches include patient education and cognitive-behavioral therapies for symptom management, which are now widely incorporated into standard healthcare practice. Thus, the complementary therapies are not necessarily distinguished from conventional therapies based on the strength of the scientific evidence. Moreover, some complementary therapies may

Table 1 Major Domains of Complementary and Alternative
Medicine*

Domain	Practices
Alternative medical systems	Traditional Chinese medicine *Techniques include: acupuncture, herbal medicine, oriental massage, Qigong* Ayurveda (traditional Indian medicine) *Treatments include: diet, exercise, meditation, herbs, massage, exposure to sunlight, controlled breathing* Homeopathic medicine *Small doses of plant extracts and minerals to stimulate the body's defense mechanisms* Naturopathic medicine *Practices include: diet and nutrition, homeopathy, acupuncture, herbal medicine, hydrotherapy, spinal and soft tissue manipulation, therapeutic counseling, pharmacology, and physical therapies involving electric currents, ultrasound, and light therapy*
Mind-body interventions	Patient education Cognitive-behavioral approaches Meditation Hypnosis Dance Music therapy Art therapy Prayer and mental healing
Biological-based therapies	Herbal therapies Special dietary therapies Orthomolecular therapies (varying combinations of chemicals) Biological therapies

(Continued)

Table 1   Major Domains of Complementary and Alternative Medicine* (*Continued*)

Domain	Practices
Manipulative and body-based methods	Chiropractic Osteopathic manipulation Massage therapy
Energy therapies	Biofield therapies *Practices include therapies intended to affect energy fields, such as Qi gong (combines movement, meditation, and controlled breathing to enhance the flow of the body's energy), Reiki (channeling spiritual energy), and Therapeutic Touch ("laying-on of hands")* Electromagnetic therapies *Involve the use of pulsed fields, magnetic fields, and alternating current or direct current fields*

*Adapted from the National Center for Complementary and Alternative Medicine website (http://nccam.nih.gov/health/whatiscam/index.htm)

become part of mainstream healthcare as studies demonstrate their effectiveness.[4–5]

Conventional healthcare has its roots in Western philosophy, is guided by scientific methods and focuses on treatment of disease. In contrast, complementary therapies often are embedded in Eastern philosophical traditions, guided by a holistic approach, and focused on the human experience of illness and wellness. However, these distinctions are not precise. Many providers of conventional healthcare, including nurses and physicians, approach the client from a holistic perspective, incorporate psychosocial therapies, and recognize the importance of provider-client partnerships and respectful communication. These qualities do not belong only to the practitioner of complementary therapies. Likewise, not all practioners of complementary therapies are holistic in their approach. Thus, discerning the difference between conventional and complementary approaches to care often is difficult.

Nursing has long embraced the holistic approach reflected in the philosophical and theoretical underpinnings of many complementary therapies. The art and science of nursing requires that nurses address the biopsychosocial and spiritual needs of clients who are receiving nursing care. The natural fit between complementary therapeutic approaches and nursing care may be particularly strong in hospice and palliative nursing. Similar to the growing popularity of many complementary therapies, hospice and palliative care developed outside mainstream healthcare in response to consumer dissatisfaction with conventional healthcare at the end of life.[5] There also is a mutual emphasis in both complementary therapies and hospice/palliative care on chronic conditions for which there is no cure, on symptom management, and on enhanced quality of life.[5] Because complementary therapies may be particularly effective in managing symptoms and promoting wellness at the end of life, hospice and palliative nurses need to be fully informed regarding many types of complementary therapies and the implications of incorporating these therapies into comprehensive care at the end of life.

Nursing roles include providing information to assist clients in making decisions about complementary therapies; understanding and communicating to others how complementary therapies affect mainstream healthcare; being knowledgeable about specific types of complementary therapies; making appropriate referrals to complementary therapists; providing some types of complementary therapies as part of standard nursing care; acquiring additional training to administer specific therapies; and conducting and disseminating research about complementary therapies.

Nurses play a central role in assisting clients in making decisions about all types of therapies, including complementary therapies. Client decisions should be based on accurate answers to the following questions:

- What are the specific goals of the therapy—cure, palliation of symptoms, avoidance of side effects from other therapy? Is there scientific evidence that the therapy is effective in achieving the stated goals?
- What are the expected benefits from this therapy?
- What are the risks, if any, associated with the therapy?
- What is the nature, prevalence and severity of side effects from this therapy?
- Does this therapy interfere with or augment the effects of other therapy that the client might be receiving?
- What are the financial costs of the therapy? Are any or all of the costs covered by the client's insurance?
- What are the qualifications of the practitioner? If appropriate, is the practitioner certified and/or licensed? Does the practitioner carry malpractice insurance?
- Is the client receiving the therapy as part of a clinical trial? If so, who is funding the trial? Has human subjects approval been obtained?

Although a number of complementary practitioners are regulated, many are not; therefore, nurses need to be familiar with any legislative and regulatory issues that could affect clients' decisions about receiving care from complementary therapy practitioners.[7]

Another important role for nurses is the incorporation of complementary therapies into their practice. Basic nursing education provides the expertise to provide some therapies such as client education. Current nursing education is insufficient, however, to prepare nurses to practice many types of complementary therapies. In some cases, basic educational requirements to ensure safe and competent practice have not been established.[6] Moreover, most state nurse practice acts currently do not provide sufficient guidance regarding nurses' roles and responsibilities in providing complementary therapies.[8,9] Despite the lack of clarity regarding nursing practice and complemen-tary therapies, nurses must seek to obtain appropriate education and credentialing in order to practice within the scope of their licensure.

The growing interest in complementary therapies also has led to increased federal and private funding to study the safety and efficacy of these treatments. One major development was the establishment in 1998 of the NCCAM as part of the NIH. The mission of the NCCAM is to stimulate, develop, and support research on CAM. Other governmental and private funding agencies also support this research. Nurses in many settings play an important role in designing, conducting, and participating in research on complementary and conventional therapies. In their role as educators and advocates, nurses also communicate research findings to clients and the public.

POSITION STATEMENT

The Hospice and Palliative Nurses Association (HPNA) is committed to a comprehensive model of care that addresses physical, emotional, and spiritual concerns of persons at the end of life through the use of conventional and complementary therapies. It is the position of the HPNA Board of Directors to:

- Acknowledge the increasing use of complementary therapies and recognize that this trend has important implications for nursing practice, education, and research.
- Recognize that many complementary therapies provide a holistic approach to managing symptoms and promoting wellness at the end of life. The holistic approach is consistent with nursing's historical and philosophical approach to practice.
- Recognize the current and potential role of complementary therapies in the amelioration of symptoms and enhancement of quality of life for hospice and palliative care clients.
- Assert that hospice and palliative nurses must possess sufficient knowledge about these therapies to guide clients in making decisions about their care and to incorporate these therapies into a comprehensive plan of care.
- Support basic and continuing nursing education focusing on complementary therapies for hospice and palliative care clients.

- Support and encourage the competent practice of complementary therapies for the purpose of promoting holistic end-of-life care.
- Affirm that some complementary therapies are within the scope of nursing practice.
- Promote regulatory and legislative clarification regarding the scope of nursing practice as it relates to complementary therapies.
- Promote increased insurance coverage for safe and effective complementary therapies.
- Encourage the conduct and dissemination of methodologically sound research that examines the efficacy, costs, and adverse effects of complementary therapies.

DEFINITION OF TERMS

Complementary and alternative medicine: "a group of diverse 'therapeutic approaches' and health care systems, practices, and products that are not presently considered to be part of conventional medicine."[2]

> *Alternative therapies:* complementary and other unconventional therapies that are used *instead* of conventional medical and surgical therapies. In contrast, *complementary therapies* are used *together with* conventional medicine.[2]
>
> A broad domain of healing resources that encompasses all health systems, modalities, and practices and their accompanying theories and beliefs, other than those intrinsic to the politically dominant health system of a particular society or culture in a given historical period. Complementary and alternative medicine (CAM) includes all such practices and ideas self-defined by their users as preventing or treating illness or promoting health and well-being. Boundaries within CAM and between the CAM domain and the domain of the dominant health system are not always sharp and fixed.[3]

Holistic nursing practice: approaches and interventions that address the needs of the whole person.[10] Holism refers to the context or philosophy of care, rather than to a set of specific therapies.[11,12]

Integrative therapies: "Integrative medicine combines mainstream medical therapies and CAM therapies for which there is some high-quality scientific evidence of safety and effectiviness."[2]

REFERENCES

1. Eisenberg DM. Trends in alternative medicine use in the United States, 1990–1997. Results of a follow-up national survey. *JAMA.* 1998;280(18):1569–1575.

2. National Center for Complementary and Alternative Medicine What is complementary and alternative medicine (CAM)? October 21, 2002. Available at: http://nccam.nih.gov/health/whatiscam/. Accessed November 6, 2002.

3. Defining and describing complementary and alternative medicine. Panel on Definition and Description, CAM Research Methodology Conference, April 1995. *Altern Ther Health Med.* 1997;3(2):49–57.

4. McAlindon TE, LaValley MP, Gulin JP, Felson DT. Glucosamine and chondroitin for treatment of osteoarthritis: A systematic quality assessment and meta-analysis. *JAMA.* 2000;283.1469–1475.

5. Pan CX. Complementary and alternative medicine in the management of pain, dyspnea, and nausea and vomiting near the end of life. A systematic review. *J Pain Symptous Manage.* 2000;20:374–387.

6. Gaydos HLB. Complementary and alternative therapies in nursing education: Trends and issues. *Online J Issues Nurs.* 2001;6(2):5.

7. Cohen MH. Legal issues in complementary and integrative medicine. A guide for the clinician. *Med Clinics North Am.* 2002;86: 185–196.

8. Sparber A. State boards of nursing and scope of practice of registered nurses performing complementary therapies. *Online J Issues Nurs* August 31, 2001 2001;6(3): Manuscript 10. Available at *http://www.nursingworld.org/ojin/topic15/tpc15_6. htm.* Accessed November 6, 2002.

9. Geddes N. Nursing and alternative medicine. Legal and practice issues. *J Holist Nurs.* 1997;15:271–281.

10. American Holistic Nurses Association. Position on the role of nurses in the practice of complementary and alternative therapies. 2002. Available at: http://www.ahna.org/about/statements. html#role. Accessed November 6, 2002

11. Frisch N. Nursing as a context for alternative/complementary modalities. *Online J Issues Nurs* May 31, 2001 2001;6(2): Manuscript 2. Available at http://www.nursingworld.org/ojin/ topic15/tpc15_2.htm). Accessed November 6, 2002.

12. Saks M. Alternative therapies: are they holistic? *Comple Therapies Nurs Midwifery.* 1997;3(1):4–8.

Approved by the HPNA Board of Directors November 2002

To obtain copies of HPNA Position statements, contact the National Office at
Penn Center West One, Suite 229, Pittsburgh, PA 15276
Phone (412) 787-9301
Fax (412) 787-9305
Website www.HPNA.org

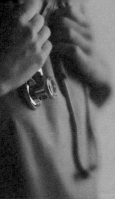

HPNA POSITION STATEMENT ON SPIRITUAL CARE

BACKGROUND

HPNA has developed this position statement to emphasize to healthcare systems and caregivers the importance of acknowledging and supporting the patient's and family's spiritual beliefs and expressions. The purpose of this position statement is to highlight the often under recognized need for spiritual support.

Spirituality is by nature and in expression, individual. It encompasses universal human needs and often includes an abiding belief in the potential of the human spirit. Spirituality may or may not include specific religious beliefs. It provides a philosophy or outlook that guides choices. It may or may not include desired outcomes such as salvation or ordination that are associated with some formal religions. There are many avenues into spiritual dimensions. Spirituality may be what gives a person strength and comfort and may become a more important concern as death approaches. It can hold a profoundly transformative potential for patients and caregivers.

Spiritual care involves the interdisciplinary team in assessing and responding to the spiritual and religious issues that concern patients and families. Spiritual care requires assessment and monitoring of a variety of aspects of the person and family and may include life review, hopes, fears, purpose and meaning, guilt and forgiveness and beliefs about afterlife.

Spiritual care values the uniqueness of each person by recognizing and honoring an individual's beliefs, values, practices and rituals and being fully open to their full discussion, expression and experience. It addresses issues of life completion in a manner consistent with the terminally ill patient's cultural and religious values and spiritual needs. Patients and families are encouraged to display their own spiritual and religious symbols and should be able to practice their own spiritual and religious rituals in an accepting atmosphere. The use of religious symbols by staff or institutions should be sensitive to cultural and religious diversity.

Spiritual distress may be expressed as or magnify the intensity of physical symptoms. Spiritual distress may occur when the individual is faced with challenges that threaten one's beliefs, meaning or purpose.

Spiritual care necessitates the ability of the caregiver to reflect on and recognize the importance of one's own spirituality and acceptance of the validity of others' spiritual beliefs. **One's own values cannot be imposed on patients and families.**

Spiritual care requires both an appreciation of the value of presence and a willingness to be fully present in providing spiritual care. Staff members need to identify their own boundaries/limitations and when there is a need for more expert assistance from chaplains or spiritual care providers. This includes attempts to notify clergy of the patient's own faith tradition, if requested.

EFFECTIVE SPIRITUAL CARE REQUIRES

- Listening actively.
- Demonstrating empathy and the ability to journey with others in their suffering.
- Recognizing and responding to another's distress and helping them to discover meaning in their experiences of suffering, grief and loss.

- Eliciting another's key concerns, including unmet spiritual and religious needs.
- Identifying and responding to ethical issues and conflicts and assisting and supporting others in the application of their own values in decision-making.
- Willingness to create therapeutic/healing spaces in which spiritual growth can occur.
- Seeking additional resources as needed by the patient including chaplaincy, other spiritual providers.

POSITION STATEMENT

The Hospice and Palliative Nurses Association (HPNA) is committed to compassionate care of persons at the end of life. It is the position of the HPNA Board of Directors to

- Acknowledge that recognition of spirituality and spiritual distress is an essential component of palliative and hospice care.
- Support *The National Consensus Project for Quality Palliative Care (NCP) Guidelines*[1] on spirituality.
- Encourage organizations to recognize and support the provision of spiritual care through education and allocation of resources.
- Commit to providing education and resources to enhance information for healthcare professionals on spirituality.
- Recognize the right of the individuals to decline spiritual care.

DEFINITION OF TERMS

Religion: a group of beliefs, a belief system or a faith tradition concerning the supernatural, sacred or divine and the moral codes, practices, values, institutions and rituals associated with such belief.[2]

    Spirituality: that which gives a person meaning, value, purpose and worth in life.

    Spiritual distress: A disturbance in the belief or value system that is a personal source of strength and hope.[3]

REFERENCES

1. Domain 5: Spiritual, Religious and Existential Aspects of Care. Clinical Practice Guidelines for Quality Palliative Care. 2004. National Consensus Project for Quality Palliative Care. Available at http://www.nationalconsensusproject.org/Guideline. Accessed February 25, 2006.
2. Religion. Wikipedia: The Free Encyclopedia. 2006. Available at http://en.wikipedia.org/wiki/religion#spirituality.   Accessed February 25, 2006.
3. Mitchell M. Problems with spiritual distress. In: Gorman LM, Raines ML, Sultan D. *Psychosocial Nursing for General patient Care.* 2nd ed. Philadelphia, PA: FA Davis: 2000:318–329.

ADDITIONAL REFERENCES

Borneman T, Brown-Saltzman K. Meaning in illness. In: Ferrell BR, Coyle N, eds. *Textbook of Palliative Nursing.* 2nd ed. New York, NY: Oxford University Press; 2006:605–615.

Kemp C. Spiritual care interventions. In: Ferrell BR, Coyle N, eds. *Textbook of Palliative Nursing.* 2nd ed. New York, NY: Oxford University Press; 2006:595–604.

Mitchell D, Gordon T. Spiritual and Religious Care Competencies for Specialist Palliative Care. Marie Curie Cancer Center. London, England. Supported by the Association of Palliative Care Chaplains. Available at www.mariecurie.org.uk/healthcare. Accessed February 25, 2006.

Neimark J. The character of happiness. *Spirituality & Health.* 2005; October:57–59.

Sing KD. Spiritual competency: an open letter to hospice colleagues. *Am J Hosp Pallia Care.* 1999; 16(4):616–618.

Taylor EJ. Spirituality and spiritual nurture in cancer care. In: Carroll-Johnson RM, Gorman LM, Bush NJ, eds. *Psychosocial Nursing Care along the Cancer Continuum.* 2nd ed. Pittsburgh, PA: Oncology Nursing Press, Inc.; 2006:117–131.

Taylor EJ. Spiritual assessment. In: Ferrell BR, Coyle N, eds. *Textbook of Palliative Nursing.* 2nd ed. New York, NY: Oxford University Press; 2006:581–594.

Approved by the HPNA Board of Directors October, 2006

To obtain copies of HPNA Position Statements, contact the National Office at
One Penn Center West, Suite 229, Pittsburgh, PA 15276-0100
Phone (412) 787-9301
Fax (412) 787-9305
Website www.HPNA.org

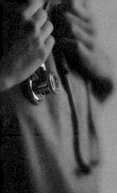

MEDICARE HOSPICE BENEFIT

HOW DOES HOSPICE WORK?

Your doctor and the hospice medical team will work with you and your family to set up a plan of care that meets your needs. Your plan of care includes hospice services that are covered by Medicare. For more specific information on a hospice plan of care, call your state or national hospice organization.

If you qualify for hospice care, you will have a specially trained medical team and support staff available to help you and your family cope with your illness. Hospice comfort care helps you make the most of the last months of life. Hospice comfort care includes use of drugs for symptom control and pain relief, physical care, counseling, equipment, and supplies to make you as comfortable and pain free as possible. **The focus of hospice is on care, not cure.**

Those involved in your care include

- you,
- your family,
- a doctor,
- a nurse,
- counselors,
- a social worker,

Medicare Hospice Benefit (http://www.medicare.gov/publications/pubs/pdf/02154.pdf)

- speech-language therapists,
- home health aides,
- homemakers, and
- volunteers.

In addition, a hospice nurse and doctor are on call 24 hours a day, seven days a week to give you and your family support and care when you need it.

Although a hospice doctor is part of the medical team, your regular doctor can also be part of this team. If you choose, a nurse practitioner may serve as your attending doctor. However, only your doctor and the hospice medical director can certify that you are terminally ill and have six months or less to live.

The hospice benefit allows you and your family to stay together in the comfort of your home. If you should need care for your illness in an inpatient hospice facility, hospital, or nursing home, the hospice medical team will make the arrangements for your stay.

WHAT WILL MEDICARE PAY FOR?

The care you get for your terminal illness must be from a **Medicare-approved** hospice program.

You can receive a one-time-only hospice consultation with a hospice medical director or hospice physician to discuss your care options and management of pain and symptoms. You don't need to choose hospice care to take advantage of this consultation service.

Medicare pays for these hospice services for your terminal illness and related conditions:

- Doctor services
- Nursing care
- Medical equipment (such as wheelchairs or walkers)

- Medical supplies (such as bandages and catheters)
- Drugs for symptom control or pain relief (you may need to pay a small copayment)
- Home health aide and homemaker services
- Physical and occupational therapy
- Speech therapy
- Social worker services
- Dietary counseling
- Grief and loss counseling for you and your family
- Short-term inpatient care
- Short-term respite care (you may need to pay a small copayment)
- Any other covered Medicare services needed to manage your pain and other symptoms, as recommended by your hospice team

---

Important:
Medicare will still pay for covered benefits for any health problems that aren't related to your terminal illness.

What is respite care?

Respite care is care given to a hospice patient by another caregiver so that the usual caregiver can rest. While in hospice care you may have one person who takes care of you every day, such as a family member. Sometimes this person needs someone to take care of you for a short time when he or she needs a break from care giving. During a period of respite care, you will be cared for in a Medicare-approved facility, such as a hospice inpatient facility, hospital, or nursing home.

WHAT WON'T MEDICARE PAY FOR?

When you choose hospice care, Medicare won't pay for any of the following:

- **Treatment intended to cure your terminal illness**

  You should talk with your doctor if you are thinking about getting treatment to cure your illness. As a hospice patient, you always have the right to stop getting hospice care at any time and receive the Medicare coverage you had before you chose hospice care.

- **Prescription drugs to cure your illness rather than for symptom control or pain relief. If you are enrolled in Medicare prescription drug coverage, however, drugs unrelated to your illness would be covered (for instance, if you needed medicine to treat an infection unrelated to your terminal illness).**

For more information about Medicare prescription drug coverage, visit www.medicare.gov on the web or call 1-800-MEDICARE (1-800-633-4227). TTY users should call 1-877-486-2048.

- **Care from any provider that wasn't set up by the hospice medical team**

  You must get hospice care from the hospice provider you chose. All care that you get for your terminal illness must be given by or arranged by the hospice medical team. You can't get the same type of hospice care from a different provider, unless you change your hospice provider.

- **Room and board**

  Room and board aren't covered by Medicare if you get hospice care in your home or if you live in a nursing home or a hospice residential facility. However, if the hospice medical team determines that you need short-term inpatient or respite services that they arrange, your stay in the facility is covered. You may be required to pay a small copayment for the respite stay.

- **Care in an emergency room, unless it's arranged by your hospice medical team**

- Care in an in-patient facility, unless it's arranged by your medical team
- Ambulance transportation, unless it's arranged by your medical team

WHAT WILL I HAVE TO PAY FOR HOSPICE CARE?

Medicare pays the hospice provider for your hospice care. You will have to pay the following:

- No more than $5 for each prescription drug and other similar products for pain relief and symptom control
- Five percent of the Medicare payment amount for inpatient respite care.

For example, if Medicare pays $ 100 per day for in-patient respite care, you will pay $5 per day. You can stay in a Medicare-approved hospital or nursing home up to five days each time you get respite care. There is no limit to the number of times you can get respite care. The amount you pay for respite care can change each year.

HOW WOULD CARE FOR A CONDITION OTHER THAN TERMINAL ILLNESS BE COVERED?

You should continue to use your Medicare plan (such as the Original Medicare Plan or a Medicare Advantage Plan) to get care for any health problems that aren't related to your terminal illness. You may be able to get this care from the hospice medical team doctor or from your own doctor. The hospice medical team must determine that any other medical care you need that isn't related to your terminal illness won't affect your care under the hospice benefit.

If you use the Original Medicare Plan, you must pay the deductible and coinsurance amounts. If you use a Medicare

Advantage Plan, you must pay the copayment. You must also continue to pay Medicare premiums, if necessary.

For more information about Medicare health plans, including deductibles, coinsurance, and copayments, look in your "Medicare & You" handbook (CMS Pub. No. 10050). If you don't have the "Medicare & You" handbook, you can get a free copy by calling 1-800-MEDICARE (1-800-633-4227). TTY users should call 1-877-486-2048. You can order the handbook online at www.medicare.gov on the web.

IMPORTANT INFORMATION ABOUT MEDIGAP (MEDICARE SUPPLEMENT INSURANCE) POLICIES

If you are in the Original Medicare Plan, you might have a Medigap policy. Your Medigap policy still helps to cover the costs for the care of health problems that aren't related to your terminal illness. Call your Medigap insurance company for more information. You can also get a free copy of "Choosing a Medigap Policy: A Guide to Health Insurance for People With Medicare" (CMS Pub. No. 02110). This guide will give you more information on using Medigap policies. To order, visit www.medicare.gov or call 1-800-MEDICARE (1-800-633-4227). TTY users should call 1-877-486-2048.

HOW LONG CAN I GET HOSPICE CARE?

You can get hospice care as long as your doctor and the hospice medical director or other hospice doctor certify that you are terminally ill and probably have six months or less to live if the disease runs its normal course. If you live longer than six months, you can still get hospice care, as long as the hospice medical director or other hospice doctor recertifies that you are terminally ill.

Important: Hospice care is given in **periods of care.** You can get hospice care for two 90-day periods followed by an unlimited number of 60-day periods. **At the start of each period of care, the hospice medical director or other hospice doctor must recertify that you are terminally ill, so that you may continue to get hospice care.** A period of care starts the day you begin to get hospice care. It ends when your 90-day or 60-day period ends.

WHY WOULD I STOP GETTING HOSPICE CARE?

If your health improves or your illness goes into remission, you no longer need hospice care. Also, you always have the right to stop getting hospice care for any reason. If you stop your hospice care, you will receive the type of Medicare coverage that you had before you chose a hospice program. If you are eligible, you can go back to hospice care at any time.

Example: Mrs. Jones has terminal cancer and received hospice care for two 90-day periods of care. Her cancer went into remission. At the start of her 60-day period of care, Mrs. Jones and her doctor decided that, due to her remission, she wouldn't need to return to hospice care at that time. Mrs. Jones' doctor told her that if she becomes eligible for hospice services in the future, she may be recertified and can return to hospice care.

CAN I CHANGE THE HOSPICE PROVIDER THAT I GET CARE FROM?

You have the right to change providers only once during each period of care.

HOW CAN I FIND A HOSPICE PROGRAM?

To find a hospice program, call your state hospice organization. The hospice program you choose must be Medicare approved to get Medicare payment. To find out if a hospice program is Medicare approved, ask your doctor, the hospice program, your state hospice organization, or your state health department.

WHERE CAN I GET MORE INFORMATION?

1. Call your state hospice organization to find a hospice program in your area.
2. Call national hospice associations or visit their Websites.
   - National Hospice and Palliative Care Organization (NHPCO)
     1700 Diagonal Road, Suite 625
     Alexandria, VA 22314
     1-800-658-8898
     www.nhpco.org
   - Hospice Association of America
     228 7th Street, SE Washington, DC 20003
     1-202-546-4759
     www.hospice-america.org
3. Visit www.medicare.gov on the web.
4. Call 1-800-MEDICARE (1-800-633-4227).
   TTY users should call 1-877-486-2048.

Note: At the time of printing, these telephone numbers were correct. Telehone numbers sometimes change. To get the most updated telephone numbers, call 1-800-MEDICARE (1-800-633-4227). TTY users should call 1-877-486-2048. Or, visit www.medicare.gov on the web. Select "Search Tools" at the top of the page.

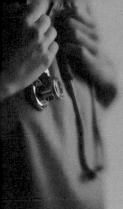

Appendix J
BREATHING PATTERNS

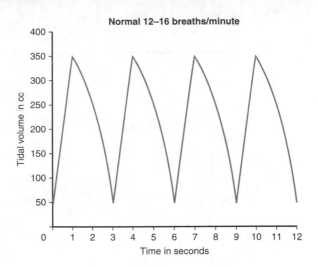

Normal 12–16 breaths/minute

Breathing patterns

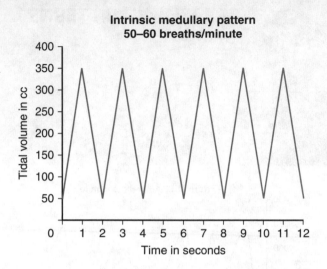

**Intrinsic medullary pattern
50–60 breaths/minute**

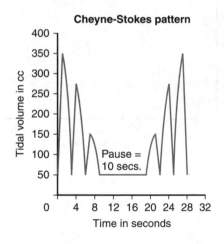

Cheyne-Stokes pattern

Pause = 10 secs.

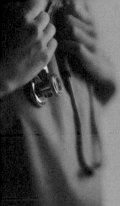

Appendix K

HOSPITAL CONDITIONS OF PARTICIPATION ABOUT ORGAN/TISSUE DONATION

A-0369

§482.45 Condition of Participation: Organ, Tissue and Eye Procurement

A-0370

§482.45(a) Standard: Organ Procurement Responsibilities

The hospital must have and implement written protocols that:

Interpretive Guidelines §482.45(a)

The hospital must have written policies and procedures to address its organ procurement responsibilities.

A-0371

§482.45(a)(1) Incorporate an agreement with an Organ Procurement Organization (OPO) designated under part 486 of this chapter, under which it must notify, in a timely manner, the

---

Hospital Conditions of Participation about Organ/Tissue Donation (http://www.cms.hhs.gov/manuals/downloads/som107ap_a_hospitals.pdf, pp. 80–88.)

OPO or a third party designated by the OPO of individuals whose death is imminent or who have died in the hospital. The OPO determines medical suitability for organ donation and, in the absence of alternative arrangements by the hospital, the OPO determines medical suitability for tissue and eye donation, using the definition of potential tissue and eye donor and the notification protocol developed in consultation with the tissue and eye banks identified by the hospital for this purpose;

Interpretive Guidelines §482.45(a)(1)

The hospital must have a written agreement with an OPO, designated under 42 CFR Part 486. At a minimum, the written agreement must address the following:

- The criteria for referral, including the referral of all individuals whose death is imminent or who have died in the hospital;
- Includes a definition of "imminent death";
- Includes a definition of "timely notification";
- Addresses the OPO's responsibility to determine medical suitability for organ donation;
- Specifies how the tissue and/or eye bank will be notified about potential donors using notification protocols developed by the OPO in consultation with the hospital-designated tissue and eye bank(s);
- Provides for notification of each individual death in a timely manner to the OPO (or designated third party) in accordance with the terms of the agreement;
- Ensures that the designated requestor training program offered by the OPO has been developed in cooperation with the tissue bank and eye bank designated by the hospital;
- Permits the OPO, tissue bank, and eye bank access to the hospital's death record information according to a designated schedule, e.g., monthly or quarterly;
- Includes that the hospital is not required to perform credentialing reviews for, or grant privileges to, members of organ

recovery teams as long as the OPO sends only **"qualified, trained individuals"** to perform organ recovery; and

- The interventions the hospital will utilize to maintain potential organ donor patients so that the patient's organs remain viable.

Hospitals must notify the OPO of every death or imminent death in the hospital. When death is imminent, the hospital must notify the OPO both before a potential donor is removed from a ventilator and while the potential donor's organs are still viable. The hospital should have a written policy, developed in coordination with the OPO and approved by the hospital's medical staff and governing body, to define "imminent death." The definition for "imminent death" should strike a balance between the needs of the OPO and the needs of the hospital's caregivers to continue treatment of a patient until brain death is declared or the patient's family has made the decision to withdraw supportive measures. Collaboration between OPOs and hospitals will create a partnership that furthers donation, while respecting the perspective of hospital staff.

The definition for "imminent death" might include a patient with severe, acute brain injury who:

- Requires mechanical ventilation;
- Is in an intensive care unit (ICU) or emergency department; **AND**
- Exhibits clinical findings consistent with a Glasgow Coma Score (GCS) that is less than or equal to a mutually-agreed-upon threshold; **or**
- MD/DOs are evaluating a diagnosis of brain death; **or**
- An MD/DO has ordered that life sustaining therapies be withdrawn, pursuant to the family's decision.

Hospitals and their OPO should develop a definition of "imminent death" that includes specific triggers for notifying the OPO about an imminent death.

In determining the appropriate threshold for the GCS, it is important to remember that if the threshold is too low, there may be too many "premature" deaths or situations where there is a loss of organ viability. Standards for appropriate GCS thresholds may be obtained from the hospital's OPO or organizations such as The Association of Organ Procurement Organizations.

Note that a patient with "severe, acute brain injury" is not always a trauma patient. For example, post myocardial infarction resuscitation may result in a patient with a beating heart and no brain activity.

The definition agreed to by the hospital and the OPO may include all of the elements listed above or just some of the elements. The definition should be tailored to fit the particular circumstances in each hospital.

Hospitals may not use "batch reporting" for deaths by providing the OPO with periodic lists of patient deaths, even if instructed to do so by the OPO. If the patient dies during a transfer from one hospital to another, it is the receiving hospital's responsibility to notify the OPO.

"Timely notification" means a hospital must contact the OPO by telephone as soon as possible after an individual has died, has been placed on a ventilator due to a severe brain injury, or who has been declared brain dead (ideally within 1 hour). That is, a hospital must notify the OPO while a brain dead or severely brain-injured, ventilator-dependent individual is still attached to the ventilator and as soon as possible after the death of any other individual, including a potential non-heart-beating donor. Even if the hospital does not consider an individual who is not on a ventilator to be a potential donor, the hospital must call the OPO as soon as possible after the death of that individual has occurred.

Referral by a hospital to an OPO is timely if it is made:

• As soon as it is anticipated that a patient will meet the criteria for imminent death agreed to by the OPO and hospital or as soon as possible after a patient meets the criteria for imminent death agreed to by the OPO and the hospital (ideally, within one hour); **AND**

• Prior to the withdrawal of any life sustaining therapies (i.e., medical or pharmacologic support).

Whenever possible, referral should be made early enough to allow the OPO to assess the patient's suitability for organ donation before brain death is declared and before the option of organ donation is presented to the family of the potential donor. Timely assessment of the patient's suitability for organ donation increases the likelihood that the patient's organs will be viable for transplantation (assuming there is no disease process identified by the OPO that would cause the organs to be unsuitable), assures that the family is approached only if the patient is medically suitable for organ donation, and assures that an OPO representative is available to collaborate with the hospital staff in discussing donation with the family.

It is the OPO's responsibility to determine medical suitability for organ donation, and, in the absence of alternative arrangements by the hospital, the OPO determines medical suitability for tissue and eye donation, using the definition of potential tissue and eye donor and the notification protocol developed in consultation with the tissue and eye banks identified by the hospital for this purpose.

Survey Procedures §482.45(a)(1)

- Review the hospital's written agreement with the OPO to verify that it addresses all required information.
- Verify that the hospital's governing body has approved the hospital's organ procurement policies.
- Review a sample of death records to verify that the hospital has implemented its organ procurement policies.
- Interview the staff to verify that they are aware of the hospital's policies and procedures for organ, tissue and eye procurement.
- Verify that the organ, tissue and eye donation program is integrated into the hospital's QAPI program.

A-0372

§482.45(a)(2) Incorporate an agreement with at least one tissue bank and at least one eye bank to cooperate in the retrieval, processing, preservation, storage and distribution of tissues and eyes, as may be appropriate to assure that all usable tissues and eyes are obtained from potential donors, insofar as such an agreement does not interfere with organ procurement;

Interpretative Guidelines §482.45(a)(2)

The hospital must have an agreement with at least one tissue bank and at least one eye bank. The OPO may serve as a "gate-keeper" receiving notification about every hospital death and should notify the tissue bank or eye bank chosen by the hospital about potential tissue and eye donors.

It is not necessary for a hospital to have a separate agreement with a tissue bank if it has an agreement with its OPO to provide tissue procurement services; nor is it necessary for a hospital to have a separate agreement with an eye bank if its OPO provides eye procurement services. The hospital is not required to use the OPO for tissue or eye procurement but is free to have an agreement with the tissue bank or eye bank of its choice. The tissue banks and eye banks define "usable tissues" and "usable eyes."

The requirements of this regulation may be satisfied through a single agreement with an OPO that provides services for organ, tissue and eye, or by a separate agreement with another tissue and/or eye bank outside the OPO, chosen by the hospital. The hospital may continue current successful direct arrangements with tissue and eye banks as long as the direct arrangement does not interfere with organ procurement.

Survey Procedures §482.45(a)(2)

Verify that the hospital has an agreement with at least one tissue bank and one eye bank that specifies criteria for referral of all potential tissue and eye donors, or an agreement with an OPO that specifies the tissue bank and eye bank to which referrals will be made. The agreement should also acknowledge that it is the OPO's responsibility to determine medical suitability for tissue and eye donation, unless the hospital has an alternative agreement with a different tissue and/or eye bank.

A-0373

§482.45(a)(3) Ensure, in collaboration with the designated OPO, that the family of each potential donor is informed of its options to donate organs, tissues, or eyes, or to decline to donate.

Interpretive Guidelines §482.45(a)(3)

It is the responsibility of the OPO to screen for medical suitability in order to select potential donors. Once the OPO has selected a potential donor, that person's family must be informed of the family's donation options.

Ideally, the OPO and the hospital will decide together how and by whom the family will be approached.

Survey Procedures §482.45(a)(3)

- Verify that the hospital ensures that the family of each potential donor is informed of its options to donate organs, tissues, or eyes, including the option to decline to donate.
- Does the hospital have QAPI mechanisms in place to ensure that the families of all potential donors are informed of their options to donate organs, tissues, or eyes, or to decline to donate?

A-0374

§482.45(a)(3) continued

The individual designated by the hospital to initiate the request to the family must be an organ procurement representative or a designated requestor. A designated requestor is an individual who has completed a course offered or approved by the OPO and designed in conjunction with the tissue and eye bank community in the methodology for approaching potential donor families and requesting organ or tissue donation;

Interpretive Guidelines §482.45(a)(3)

The individual designated by the hospital to initiate the request to a family must be an organ procurement representative, an **organizational representative of a tissue or eye bank,** or a designated requestor. Any individuals involved in a request for organ, tissue, and eye donation must be formally trained in the donation request process.

The individual designated by the hospital to initiate the request to the family must be an OPO, tissue bank, or eye bank representative or a designated requestor. A **"designated requestor"** is defined as a hospital-designated individual who has completed a course offered or approved by the OPO and designed in conjunction with the tissue and eye bank community.

Ideally, the OPO and the hospital will decide together how and by whom the family will be approached. If possible, the OPO representative and a designated requestor should approach the family together.

The hospital must ensure that any "designated requestor" for organs, tissues or eyes has completed a training course either offered or approved by the OPO, which addresses methodology for approaching potential donor families.

Survey Procedures §482.45(a)(3)

- Review training schedules and personnel files to verify that all designated requestors have completed the required training.
- How does the hospital ensure that only OPO, tissue bank, or eye bank staff or designated requestors are approaching families to ask them to donate?

A-0375

§482.45(a)(4) Encourage discretion and sensitivity with respect to the circumstances, views, and beliefs of the families of potential donors;

Interpretive Guidelines §482.45(a)(4)

Using discretion does not mean a judgment can be made by the hospital that certain families should not be approached about donation. Hospitals should approach the family with the belief that a donation is possible and should take steps to ensure the family is treated with respect and care. The hospital staff's perception that a family's grief, race, ethnicity, religion or socioeconomic background would prevent donation should never be used as a reason not to approach a family.

All potential donor families must be approached and informed of their donation rights.

Survey Procedures §482.45(a)(4)

- Interview a hospital-designated requestor regarding approaches to donation requests.
- Review the designated requestor training program to verify that it addresses the use of discretion.
- Review the hospital's complaint file for any relevant complaints.

A-0376

§482.45(a)(5) Ensure that the hospital works cooperatively with the designated OPO, tissue bank and eye bank in educating staff on donation issues;

Interpretive Guidelines §482.45(a)(5)

Appropriate hospital staff, including all patient care staff, must be trained on donation issues. The training program must be developed in cooperation with the OPO, tissue bank and eye bank, and should include, at a minimum:

- Consent process;
- Importance of using discretion and sensitivity when approaching families;
- Role of the designated requestor;

- Transplantation and donation, including pediatrics, if appropriate;
- Quality improvement activities; and
- Role of the organ procurement organization.

Training should be conducted with new employees annually, whenever there are policy/procedure changes, or when problems are determined through the hospital's QAPI program.

Those hospital staff who may have to contact or work with the OPO, tissue bank and eye bank staff must have appropriate training on donation issues including their duties and roles.

Survey Procedures §482.45(a)(5)

- Review in-service training schedules and attendance sheets.
- How does the hospital ensure that all appropriate staff has attended an educational program regarding donation issues and how to work with the OPO, tissue bank, and eye bank?

A-0377

§482.45(a)(5) continued

Reviewing death records to improve identification of potential donors; and

Interpretive Guidelines §482.45(a)(5)

Hospitals must cooperate with the OPOs, tissue banks and eye banks in regularly or periodically reviewing death records. This means that the hospital must develop policies and procedures which permit the OPO, tissue bank, and eye bank access to death record information that will allow the OPO, tissue bank and eye bank to assess the hospital's donor potential, assure that all deaths or imminent deaths are being referred to the OPO in a timely manner, and identify areas where the hospital, OPO, tissue bank and eye bank staff performance might be improved. The policies must address how patient confidentiality will be maintained during the review process.

Survey Procedures §482.45(a)(5)

- Verify by review of policies and records that the hospital works with the OPO, tissue bank, and eye bank in reviewing death records.
- Verify that the effectiveness of any protocols and policies is monitored as part of the hospital's quality improvement program.
- Validate how often the reviews are to occur. Review the protocols that are in place to guide record reviews and analysis.
- Determine how confidentiality is ensured.

A-0378

§482.45(a)(5) continued

Maintaining potential donors while necessary testing and placement of potential donated organs, tissues, and eyes take place.

Interpretive Guidelines §482.45(a)(5)

The hospital must have policies and procedures, developed in cooperation with the OPO, that ensure that potential donors are maintained in a manner that maintains the viability of their organs. The hospital must have policies in place to ensure that potential donors are identified and declared dead within an acceptable time frame by an appropriate practitioner.

Survey Procedures §482.45(a)(5)

- Determine by review, what policies and procedures are in place to ensure that potential donors are identified and declared dead by an appropriate practitioner within an acceptable timeframe.
- Verify that there are policies and procedures in place to ensure the coordination between facility staff and OPO staff in maintaining the potential donor.

A-0379

§482.45(b) Standard: Organ Transplantation Responsibilities

1. A hospital in which organ transplants are performed must be a member of the Organ Procurement and Transplantation Network (OPTN) established and operated in accordance with section 372 of the Public Health Service (PHS) Act (42 U.S.C. 274) and abide by its rules. The term "rules of the OPTN" means those rules provided for in regulations issued by the secretary in accordance with section 372 of the PHS Act which are enforceable under 42 CFR 121.10. No hospital is considered to be out of compliance with section 1138(a)(1)(B) of the Act, or with the requirements of this paragraph, unless the secretary has given the OPTN formal notice that he or she approves the decision to exclude the hospital from the OPTN and has notified the hospital in writing.

2. For purposes of these standards, the term "organ" means a human kidney, liver, heart, lung, or pancreas.

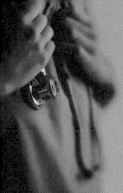

Edmonton Symptom Scale. Reproduced, with permission, *Journal of Palliative Care*.

Site Number (Assigned) —————

Patient ID —————   Date of Initial Consult ___ / ___ / ___

	Day 1	Day 2	Day 3	Day 4	Day 5	Day 6	Day 7	Day 8	Day 9	Day 10	Day 11	Day 12	Day 13	Day 14	Day 15
Date (month/day)															
Symptom															
Pain															
Tiredness (Fatigue)															
Drowsiness (Sleepiness)															
Depression															
Anxiety															
Nausea															
Anorexia															
Shortness of Breath															
Secretions (Y/N)															
Constipation (Y/N)															
Unable to Respond (Y/N)															
Delirium (Y/N)															
ASSESSED BY:	P F T	P F T	P F T	P F T	P F T	P F T	P F T	P F T	P F T	P F T	P F T	P F T	P F T	P F T	P F T
Completion Code															

Assessment Scale:	None = 0	Mild = 1	Moderate = 2*	Severe* = 3	*Requires daily follow-up, plus 72 hour follow-up
Completion Code:	Completed = 1	Not Completed, not seen/patient died/signed off = 2		Not Completed Other Reason = 3	

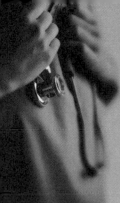

Appendix M

MEMORIAL SYMPTOM ASSESSMENT SCALE

Memorial Symptom Scale.(Reprinted from *European Journal of Cancer,* 30, Portenoy RK et al., The Memorial Symptom Assessment Scale, 1326–1336, 1994, with permission from Elsevier.)

Name									Date				

Section 1

Instructions: We have listed 24 symptoms below. Read each one carefully. If you have had the symptom during this past week, let us know how <u>OFTEN</u> you had it, how <u>SEVERE</u> it was usually and how much it <u>DISTRESSED or BOTHERED</u> you by circling the appropriate number. If you <u>DID NOT HAVE</u> the symptom, make an "X" in the box marked "<u>DID NOT HAVE</u>."

DURING THE PAST WEEK Did you have any of the following symptoms?	D I D N O T H A V E	IF YES How OFTEN did you have it?				IF YES How SEVERE was it usually				IF YES How much did it DISTRESS or BOTHER you?				
		Rarely	Occasionally	Frequently	Almost Constantly	Slight	Moderate	Severe	Very Severe	Not at all	A Little Bit	Somewhat	Quite a Bit	Very Much
Difficulty concentrating		1	2	3	4	1	2	3	4	0	1	2	3	4
Pain		1	2	3	4	1	2	3	4	0	1	2	3	4
Lack of energy		1	2	3	4	1	2	3	4	0	1	2	3	4
Cough		1	2	3	4	1	2	3	4	0	1	2	3	4
Feeling nervous		1	2	3	4	1	2	3	4	0	1	2	3	4
Dry mouth		1	2	3	4	1	2	3	4	0	1	2	3	4
Nausea		1	2	3	4	1	2	3	4	0	1	2	3	4
Feeling drowsy		1	2	3	4	1	2	3	4	0	1	2	3	4
Numbness/tingling in hands/feet		1	2	3	4	1	2	3	4	0	1	2	3	4
Difficulty sleeping		1	2	3	4	1	2	3	4	0	1	2	3	4
Feeling bloated		1	2	3	4	1	2	3	4	0	1	2	3	4
Problems with urination		1	2	3	4	1	2	3	4	0	1	2	3	4
Vomiting		1	2	3	4	1	2	3	4	0	1	2	3	4
Shortness of breath		1	2	3	4	1	2	3	4	0	1	2	3	4
Diarrhea		1	2	3	4	1	2	3	4	0	1	2	3	4
Feeling sad		1	2	3	4	1	2	3	4	0	1	2	3	4
Sweats		1	2	3	4	1	2	3	4	0	1	2	3	4
Worrying		1	2	3	4	1	2	3	4	0	1	2	3	4
Problems with sexual interest or activity		1	2	3	4	1	2	3	4	0	1	2	3	4
Itching		1	2	3	4	1	2	3	4	0	1	2	3	4
Lack of appetite		1	2	3	4	1	2	3	4	0	1	2	3	4
Dizziness		1	2	3	4	1	2	3	4	0	1	2	3	4
Difficulty swallowing		1	2	3	4	1	2	3	4	0	1	2	3	4
Feeling irritable		1	2	3	4	1	2	3	4	0	1	2	3	4

Section 2									
INSTRUCTIONS: We have listed 8 symptoms below. Read each one carefully. If you have had the symptom during this past week, let us know how SEVERE it was usually and how much it DISTRESSED or BOTHERED you by circling the appropriate number. If you DID NOT HAVE the symptom, make an "X" in the box marked "DID NOT HAVE."									
DURING THE PAST WEEK, Did you have any of the following symptoms ?	D I D N O T H A V E	IF YES How SEVERE was it usually?				IF YES How much did it DISTRESS or BOTHER you?				
		Slight	Moderate	Severe	Very Severe	Not at all	A little bit	Somewhat	Quite a bit	Very much
Mouth sores		1	2	3	4	0	1	2	3	4
Change in the way food tastes		1	2	3	4	0	1	2	3	4
Weight loss		1	2	3	4	0	1	2	3	4
Hair loss		1	2	3	4	0	1	2	3	4
Constipation		1	2	3	4	0	1	2	3	4
Swelling of arms or legs		1	2	3	4	0	1	2	3	4
"I don't look like myself"		1	2	3	4	0	1	2	3	4
Changes in skin		1	2	3	4	0	1	2	3	4
IF YOU HAD ANY OTHER SYMPTOMS DURING THE PAST WEEK, PLEASE LIST BELOW AND INDICATE HOW MUCH THE SYMPTOMHAS DISTRESSED OR BOTHERED YOU.									
Other:						0	1	2	3	4
Other:						0	1	2	3	4
Other:						0	1	2	3	4

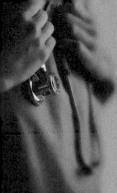

Appendix N

OPIOID REFERENCE TABLE

Opioid Reference Table.

Drug Name Available Dosage	Appropriate Opioid Equianalgesic Dose		Oral to Perenteral Dose Ratio	Dosing Interval (Hours)	Strenghts of Products mg CR: Continuous Release IR: Instant Release
	Oral (mg)	Parenteral (mg)			
Morphine	30	10	3:1	CR 12	MSContin 15,30,60,100,200mg Tablets Oramorph 15,30,60,100 mg Tablets
	30	10	3:1	IR 4	MSIR, Roxanol, RMS-Tab., Liq. Supp.
Hydromorphone	7.5	1.5	5:1	IR 4	Dilaudid 1,2,3,4 mg Tab., Liq., Supp.
Oxycodone	15	N/A	N/A	CR 12	Oxycontin 10,20,40,80 mg
					Roxicodone, OxyIR, oxyfast are brand names—Percocet and Roxicet contain a combination of oxycodone and acetaminophen. All are available in tablet or liquid form
Hydrocodone	30	N/A	N/A	N/A	Vicodin (hydrocodone bitartrate, acetaminophen) Vicodin 5 (5 mg/ 500 mg) Vicodin 7.5 (7.5 mg/750 mg) Vicodin 10 (10 mg/660 mg)
Codeine	200	130	1.5:1	N/A	15, 20, 60 mg Tablets Doses exceeding 65 mg are not recommended due to increasing constipation side effects.
Meperidine	300	75	4:1	N/A	Demerol 50, 100 mg Tablets, syrup Not recommended for administration> 48 hrs. or for cancer pain management.
Levorphanol	4	2	2:1	6–8	Levo-Dromoran 2 mg Tablets Long half-life: must be used with caution to avoid delayed accumulation.
Methadone			N/A	Variable during titration	5, 10, 40 mg Tab., Liq. Very good for neuropathic pain. Long half-life: must be used with extreme caution to avoid accumulation
Fentanyl	Refer to conversion	Refer to conversion	N/A	72 hrs.	Duragesic 25, 50, 75, 100 mcg Patch It is necessary to also use a breakthrough medication.

Principles of Administration

- WHO Ladder
  - For mild pain (unless contraindicated) use aspirin, acetaminophen or nonsteroidal anti-inflammatory agents.
  - If pain persists from mild to moderate pain use, Percocet, Tylenol #3, Vicodin or oxycodone.
  - If pain continues or becomes moderate to severe, increase the opioid (i.e. morphine, Dilaudid and Oxycontin)
- Adjuvant medications are added to medication regimen as indicated on adjuvant medication list.
- Breakthrough dose: 1/3 to 1/2 of the twelve = hour dose or 10–15% of the 24 hour dose.
- Titrating dosage:
  - A. If 3 or more breakthrough doses in a 24-hour period, re-titration of opioid is necessary.
    - Calculate increase based upon total opioid dose (ATC + Breakthrough) taken in the
  - OR previous 24-hour period.
    - Increase both the ATC and Breakthrough doses.
  - B. Use the following guideline: Pain > 7   Increase dose by 50% to 100%
         Pain 4–7   Increase dose by 25% to 50%
         Pain < 4   Increase dose by 25%
    - Once a patient has 2 or less breakthrough doses and a steadystate of medication has been reached, then a continuous release equianalgesic opioid may be initiated. Always start withan instant release before switching to continuous release.
- Switch from fixed combination opioids to a single entity opioid when acetaminophen dose> 4000 mg/day.
- Conversion equation:
$$\frac{\text{Equianalgesic dose (route)}}{\text{24 h dose (route)}} = \frac{\text{Equianalgesic dose (route)}}{\text{24 h dose (route)}}$$
current opioid   desired new opioid

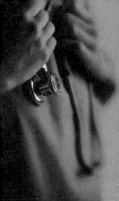

1. **Opioid heterogeneity:** Not all opioids are created equal. There are variations in
   - Metabolism
   - Potency
   - Available routes of administration
   - Toxicity
   - Side effect profile
   - Presence or absence of ceiling effect
   - Interaction with the opioid receptors in the body—referred to incomplete cross-sensitivity or incomplete cross-tolerance.

2. **Switching opioids:** It is common in clinical practice to find that it is necessary to change either the route or the drug in a patient receiving opioid analgesics. Examples include:
   - Patient has become NPO, must switch from oral to parenteral
   - Patient is transitioning from postop parenteral to a different drug given orally
   - High or escalating doses of one opioid are causing unacceptable side effects and must be changed

---

Opioid Potency and Equianalgesia. Reproduced, with permission, Tom Quinn, Massachusetts General Hospital, April 2008.

- Insurance coverage favors one drug over another
- A medication taken in the community is not on formulary in the institution

3. **Potency:** Potency refers to the amount of drug required to produce an effect. A major difference among opioids is the difference in potency: the same mg amount of one opioid will have different analgesic effects and side/toxic effects than a different opioid. When differences in potency are not taken into consideration, especially when changing routes or changing drugs, significant dosing errors can occur.

- Patient may be undermedicated and in severe pain
- Patient may be overmedicated and experience sedation' significant respiratory depression, and even death

4. **Relative potency:** Morphine 30 mg PO is the reference drug against which the others are measured. Relative potencies can be easily viewed on equianalgesic tables (see table).

5. **PO vs IV potency:** Because of differences in metabolism between oral and parenteral routes, the parenteral opioid is always more potent than the same mg amount of the oral opioid.

6. **Common potency-related errors:** The most common hospital-based source of error involving issues of potency is when a patient is switched from morphine to hydromorphone (Dilaudid). **Hydromorphone by any route is significantly more potent than morphine**

- Oral hydromorphone is 4 times more potent than oral morphine:

     7.5 mg hydromorphone PO = 30 mg morphine PO

- Parenteral hydromorphone is 7 times more potent than parenteral morphine:

     1.5 mg hydromorphone IV = 10 mg morphine IV

- Parenteral hydromorphone is 20 times more potent than oral morphine:

     1.5 mg hydromorphone IV = 30 mg morphine PO

7. **Opioid rotation:** Changing from one opioid to another is referred to as "opioid rotation" or "opioid switching."
   - Indications for switching from one opioid to another include
     - Opioid-induced intractable and intolerable side effects
     - Inadequate analgesia despite appropriate dose escalation
   - The primary goal of opioid rotation protocols is to find a safe starting dose of the new opioid
   - The regimen is then titrated to the individual patient's needs using a combination of a scheduled dose and liberal use of PRN "rescue" doses

8. **Principles of opioid rotation:** Safe opioid rotation adheres to the following principles:
   - Use a consistent method or protocol
   - Consistently use the same equianalgesic table for calculating doses (there may be slight differences from one table to another)
   - In most cases, reduce the calculated dose by a standard percentage (25–50%) to account for:
     - Incomplete cross-tolerance
     - Variations in patient metabolism
     - Limitations of equianalgesic tables
     - Reducing the calculated dose may not be necessary when route alone is being changed
   - When rounding, round downward
   - Use a PRN rescue dose of 10% of the 24-hour dose, and available q 1 hour.
   - Adjust the scheduled dose after 24 hours based on total opioid intake (scheduled + PRN) over the previous day

9. **Using an equianalgesic table:** An equianalgesic table accounts for differences in potency by providing the approximate equivalent dose by route of multiple opioids compared to morphine 30 mg PO.

- All values on an equianalgesic table represent doses that are equivalent to each other in terms of potency
- The values on the table may be used to create simple ratio equations for calculating equianalgesic doses of any drugs in the table

Opioid Equianalgesic Doses

Oral (mg)	Drug	Parenteral (mg)
30	Morphine	10
20	Oxycodone	N/A
7.5	Hydromorphone	1.5
N/A	Fentanyl	0.1 (100 mcg)
200	Codeine	130
20	Hydrocodone	N/A

Step 1: Set up the equation

Values from the table Patient opioid values Solve for X

$$\frac{\text{Value of opioid 1}}{\text{Value of opioid 2}} = \frac{\substack{\text{24-hour dose of} \\ \text{current opioid} \\ \text{(opioid 1)}}}{\substack{X \text{ amt. of new} \\ \text{opioid (opioid 2)}}} = \substack{\text{Equianalgesic} \\ \text{24-hour dose} \\ \text{of opioid 2}}$$

Step 2: Reduce calculated 24-hour dose by 25–50% = 24-hour starting dose

Step 3: Divide 24-hour starting dose by number of doses per day = scheduled dose

Step 4: Order liberal "rescue" dose (10–15% of 24-hour starting dose) and titrate to comfort

Step 5: Monitor patient closely for balance of analgesia, function, and side effects

Step 6: After 12–24 hours recalculate scheduled dose:
Total opioid in 24 hours (scheduled + rescue) ÷ doses per day = new scheduled dose

Example 1: Mr. J. is on stable dose of sustained release oral morphine' but is now NPO. He has been taking MS
Contin 60 mg q 12 hr plus 20 mg morphine solu-
tion 1–2 times per day for breakthrough pain. What
is the appropriate starting dose of IV morphine?

Values from the table	Patient opioid values	Solve for X
$\dfrac{\text{Morphine 30 mg PO}}{\text{Morphine 10 mg IV}}$	$= \dfrac{120 \text{ mg morphine PO}}{\text{morphine } X\text{mg IV}} =$	Equianalgesic 24-hour dose of opioid 2

*(Note that a conservative estimate of 24-hour intake was used and
did not include the PRN doses)*

Solve for X by cross-multiplying:
(MS 30 mg) × (X) = (MS 10 mg) × (MS 120 mg) =
30X= 1200, X = 40 mg. Divide by 24 to calculate the infusion rate = 1.6 mg/hr

Example 2: Ms A. has advanced endometrial cancer. Ms. A's
abdominal pain is well controlled (range: 0 –
3/10) with 100 mg MS Contin q8 hours. She has
a rescue dose of immediate release morphine 30
mg PO ordered' but rarely needs it. Comorbid
conditions require a change of drug and route.

Doing the math:

a. First calculate the 24 hour basal dose: morphine 100 mg ×
3 doses per day = 300 mg.

b. Set up the simple proportion equation:

Values from the table	Patient opioid values	Solve for X
$\dfrac{\text{Morphine 30 mg PO}}{\text{Dilaudid 1.5 mg IV}}$	$= \dfrac{\text{Morphine 300 mg PO}}{\text{Dilaudid } X \text{ mg IV}} =$	15 mg Dilaudid IV/24 hr

c. Reduce dose by 25%: 15 × .75 = 11.25 mg IV to be delivered
over 24 hours by continuous infusion.

d. The hourly rate is 11.25 + 24 = 0.5 mg/hour.

e. The rescue dose is 10–15% of the 24 dose: 11 × .1 = 1.1 mg.
Suggested rescue dose: 0.5 – 2 mg IV q 1 hour as needed for
breakthrough pain.

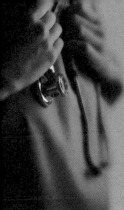

Appendix P
BENZODIAZEPINE EQUIVALENTS

I. Indications
  A. *Benzodiazepine withdrawal*
  B. *Barbiturate withdrawal*
  C. Sedative withdrawal

II. General
  A. Equivalents to 60 mg *Diazepam* or 180 mg Phenobarbital
  B. Equivalent = drug dose × conversion factor

III. Benzodiazepines equivalents to diazepam 60 mg
  A. *Alprazolam (Xanax)* 6 mg
    1. *Valium* = dose × 10
    2. Phenobarbital = dose × 30
  B. *Chlordiazepoxide (Limbitrol)* 150 mg
    1. *Valium* = dose × 0.4
    2. Phenobarbital = dose × 1.2
  C. *Clonazepam (Klonopin)* 24 mg
    1. *Valium* = dose × 2.5
    2. Phenobarbital = dose × 7.5

Benzodiazepine Equivalents. Reproduced, with permission, Moses, S. ©2008, Family Practice Notebook LLC. http://www.fpnotebook.com/PSY53.htm

    D. *Flurazepam* (*Dalmane*) 90 mg
       1. *Valium* = dose × 0.6
       2. Phenobarbital = dose × 2.0
    E. *Halazepam* (*Paxipam*) 240 mg
       1. *Valium* = dose × 0.25
       2. Phenobarbital = dose × 0.75
    F. *Lorazepam* (*Ativan*) 12 mg
       1. *Valium* = dose × 5.0
       2. Phenobarbital = dose × 15.0
    G. *Oxazepam* (*Serax*) 60 mg
       1. *Valium* = dose × 1.0
       2. Phenobarbital = dose × 3.0
    H. *Temazepam* (*Restoril*) 60 mg
       1. *Valium* = dose × 1.0
       2. Phenobarbital = dose × 3.0

IV. Barbiturate equivalents to Phenobarbital 180 mg
    A. Butabarbital (Butisol) 600 mg
       1. *Valium* = dose × 0.1
       2. Phenobarbital = dose × 0.3
    B. Pentobarbital (Nembutal) 600 mg
       1. *Valium* = dose × 0.1
       2. Phenobarbital = dose × 0.3
    C. Secobarbital (Seconal) 600 mg
       1. *Valium* = dose × 0.1
       2. Phenobarbital = dose × 0.3
    D. Phenobarbital 180 mg
       1. *Valium* = dose × 0.33
       2. Phenobarbital = dose × 1.0

V. Miscellaneous sedative equivalents
    A. Glycerol: *meprobamate* (*equanil*) 2400 mg
       1. *Valium* = dose × 0.025
       2. Phenobarbital = dose × 0.075

B. Piperidinedione: glutethimide (Doriden) 1500 mg
   1. *Valium* = dose × 0.04
   2. Phenobarbital = dose × 0.12
C. Quinazoline: *methaqualone* 1800 mg
   1. *Valium* = dose × 0.03
   2. Phenobarbital = dose × 0.1

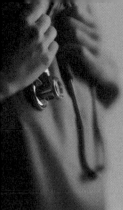

HPNA POSITION STATEMENT ON PALLIATIVE SEDATION AT END OF LIFE

BACKGROUND

Patients at the end of life may suffer an array of physical, psychological symptoms and existential distress that, in most cases, can be relieved through optimal end-of-life care. However, the suffering of some patients is intractable to such efforts. For imminently dying patients whose suffering is unrelenting and unendurable, palliative sedation may offer relief.

Palliative sedation is the monitored use of medications intended to induce varying degrees of unconsciousness, but not death, for relief of refractory and unendurable symptoms in imminently dying patents.[1–6] The prevalence of palliative sedation in clinical practice is unknown but reports suggest that it is used in 15–30% of dying patients.[5–7] Palliative sedation may also be termed terminal sedation, total sedation, sedation for intractable symptoms at end of life, continuous or prolonged sedation.[1,8] It is distinct from procedural and respite sedation.[8]

The ethical justification for palliative sedation is based in precepts of dignity, autonomy, beneficence, fidelity, nonmaleficence, and the rule of double effect. These principles endorse the right of the individual to make health care decisions based on personal values and quality of life considerations, and the responsibility of clinicians to provide humane and compassionate care that is consistent with professional and societal norms.

The use of medication to promote comfort and relieve pain in dying patients is supported by the American Nurses Association (ANA)[9] who state, "achieving adequate symptom control, even at the expense of life, thus hastening death is ethically justified." This statement is reiterated in the ANA's Code of Ethics for Nurses[10] which also states that nurses may not act with the sole intent to end a patient's life even if motivated by compassion and concern for dignity and quality of life. Thus, palliative sedation with its intent to relieve suffering in dying patients but not to deliberately hasten death is seen as distinct from euthanasia or assisted suicide where the intent is solely to end life.[11] These statements reflect the rule of double effect.

Interdisciplinary assessment of the patient to determine the refractory nature of his/her suffering and communication with the patient, family/significant other/surrogate decision maker, and other health care providers is critical to determine the appropriateness of palliative sedation and assure a valid informed consent process.

The use of palliative sedation requires that comfort be the priority goal of care. The use of cardiopulmonary resuscitation is generally viewed as inconsistent with this goal. However, decisions to withhold or withdraw other life sustaining therapies including artificial hydration and nutrition are separate from, but may be related to, the decision to use palliative sedation.[12]

POSITION STATEMENT

The Hospice and Palliative Nurses Association (HPNA) is committed to compassionate care of persons at end of life. It is the position of the HPNA Board of Directors to:

- Affirm the value of end of life care that includes aggressive and comprehensive symptom management.
- Affirm the use of palliative sedation to manage refractory and unendurable symptoms in imminently dying patients as one method of aggressive and comprehensive symptom management.

- Assert that hospice and palliative care nurses must possess sufficient knowledge about the issues surrounding the use of palliative sedation to inform patients, families, and other health care providers in making decisions about its use.

- Direct those nurses who choose not to care for patient's receiving palliative sedation to continue to provide care until responsibility for care is transferred to an equally competent colleague.

- Honor nurses rights to transfer care.

- Affirm that consultation with, psychiatry, ethicists, chaplains, social workers, pharmacists, and palliative care specialists may be needed to assure appropriateness of palliative sedation.

- Oppose active euthanasia[13] and assisted suicide[14] as a means to relieve suffering.

DEFINITION OF TERMS

Autonomy: a multidimensional ethical concept. It is the right of a capable person to decide his/her own course of action. Self-determination is a legal right.[15]

   Beneficence: an ethical duty to do well. It relates to promoting well being.[15]

   Dignity or respect for person: a fundamental ethical principle. Dignity is the quality or state or being honored or valued. Respecting the body, values, beliefs, goals, privacy, actions and priorities of an autonomous adult preserves their dignity. This is a broader concept than autonomy.[10,15,16]

   Double effect: an ethical principle based in Roman Catholic theology that is used when it is not possible to avoid all harmful effects. For an action to be ethically permissible under the principle of double effect, the act itself must be good or at least neutral (e.g., administering analgesic or sedative medication); the intention of the act is to produce a good effect (i.e., relief of suffering) even though a harmful effect (i.e., death) is foreseeable in some circumstances; the harmful effect of the act must not be the means to the good effect (i.e., death is not the means to relief of suffering); the good effect must outweigh or balance the harmful effect.[4,15]

Fidelity: the ethical imperative to keep promises. For health care providers, fidelity includes the promise not to abandon the patient.[15]

Informed consent: a tenet of autonomy. To make an informed, autonomous decision, the person must have the capacity to understand the consequences of the decision; sufficient information about the treatment, desired outcomes, foreseeable consequences; intent to make the decision without coercion.[15]

Imminent death: refers to death that is expected to occur within hours to days based on the person's current condition, progression of disease, and symptom constellation.[5,17]

Intent: the purpose or state of mind at the time of an action. Intent of the patient/ proxy and health care providers is a critical issue in ethical decision making around palliative sedation. Relief of suffering, not hastening or causing death, is the intent of palliative sedation.[4,15]

Proxy decision making: allowed if the person lacks capacity to make an informed choice. Written advanced directives, substituted judgment based on subjective knowledge of the person's values, views on quality of life, goals, or the "best interest" of the person whose wishes and values are unknown based on benefits/ burden weighing of recommended actions are the basis of such surrogate decisions.[1,15,16]

Nonmaleficence: the ethical duty to do no harm. When beneficence conflicts with nonmaleficence, there is a greater duty to avoid inflicting harm.[15,16]

Palliative sedation: the monitored use of medications intended to provide relief of refractory symptoms by inducing varying degrees of unconsciousness but not death in terminally ill patients.[1–6]

Refractory symptom: one that cannot be adequately controlled in a tolerable time frame despite aggressive use of usual therapies, and seems unlikely to be adequately controlled by further invasive or noninvasive therapies without excessive or intolerable acute or chronic side effects/complications.[2]

Respite sedation: the use of sedation for a brief, planned period to provide symptom relief and rest with the goal of returning to consciousness and pursuing future therapeutic and/or palliative therapies.[8,12,18]

Suffering: a phenomenon of conscious existence. It is an aversive emotional experience brought on by an enduring perceived or actual threat to physical, psychological, social, spiritual well-being.[19]

Withholding and withdrawing life sustaining therapy (LST): is legally and ethically permissible if it is the patient's fully informed and freely made wish; or such therapy is causing or will cause harm to the patient; or the therapy is not or will not benefit the patient in the future. Artificial hydration and nutrition may be withheld or withdrawn based on the same grounds.[16]

REFERENCES

1. National Hospice and Palliative Care Organization (NHPCO). *Total Sedation: A Hospice and Palliative Care Resource Guide.* National Hospice and Palliative Care Organization. 2001.

2. Cherny, N. & Portenoy, RK. Sedation in the management of refractory symptoms: Guidelines for evaluation and treatment. *J Pallia Care.* 1994;10:31–38.

3. Quill, TE & Byock, IR. Responding to intractable terminal suffering: The role of sedation and voluntary refusal of food and fluids. *Ann Intern Med.* 2000;132:408–414.

4. Rousseau, P. The ethical validity and clinical experience of palliative sedation. *Mayo Clinic Proceedings.* 2000;71:1064–1069.

5. Cowan, JD & Walsh, D. Terminal sedation in palliative medicine—definition and review of the literature. *Support Care Cancer.* 2001;9:403–407.

6. Beel, A; Mc Clement, SE; & Harlos M. Palliative sedation therapy: A review of definitions and usage. *Int Pallia Nur.* 2002; 8(4):190–199.

7. Cowan, JD & Palmer, TW. Practical guide to palliative sedation. *Curr Oncol Rep.* 2002;4:242–249.

8. Rousseau, P. Existential suffering and palliative sedation in terminal illness. *Progr Palliat Care.* 2002;10:222–224.

9. American Nurses Association Position Statement on Promotion of Comfort and Relief of pain in dying patients. 1991. Accessed 9/1/02 www.nursingworld.org/readroom/position/ethics/etpain.htm

10. American Nurses Association. *Code of Ethics for Nurses with Interpretive Statements.* Washington, DC American Nurses Publishing, 2001.

11. Burt, RA. The Supreme Court speaks: Not assisted suicide but a constitutional right to palliative care. *N Engl J Med.* 1997;337:1234–1236.

12. Cherny, N. The use of sedation in the management of refractory pain. *Principles & Practice of Supportive Oncology Updates.* 2000; 3(4):1–11.

13. Hospice and Palliative Nurses Association (HPNA). Position Statement: Legalization of Assisted Suicide. 2001. www.hpna. org/position suicide.asp Accessed 12/28/02.

14. American Nurses Association (ANA). Position Statement: Active euthanasia. 1994. www.nursingworld.org/readroom/position/ethics/eteuth.htm Accessed 1/30/03.

15. Beauchamp, TL & Childress, JF. *Principles of Biomedical Ethics,* 5th ed. New York: Oxford University Press, 2001.

16. Schwarz, JK. Ethical aspects of palliative care in ML Matzo & DW Sherman, eds. *Palliative Care Nursing: Quality Care to the End of Life.* New York: Springer Publishing Co.; 2001.

17. Jansen, LA & Sulmasy, DP. Sedation, alimentation, hydration and equivocation: Careful conversation about care at end of life. *Ann Inter Med,* 2002;136:845–849.

18. Fine, P. Total sedation in end of life care: Clinical considerations. *J Hosp Palliat Nur.* 2001;3(3): 81–87.

19. Cherny, NI; Coyle, N; & Foley, KM. Suffering in the advanced cancer patient: A definition and taxonomy. *J Pallia Care.* 1994;10:57–70.

Developed by:
Constance Dahlin, RN, CS, APN Maureen Lynch, MS, RN, CS, AOCN, CHPN

Approved by the HPNA Board of Directors June 2003

To obtain copies of HPNA Position Statements, contact the National Office at
Penn Center West One, Suite 229, Pittsburgh, PA 15276
Phone (412) 787-9301
Fax (412) 787-9305
Website www.HPNA.org

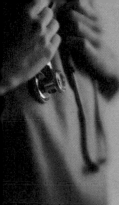

Appendix R
VENTILATOR WITHDRAWAL ALGORITHM

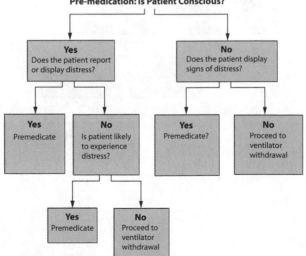

Advance Preparations
- Notify OPO
- Prepare family
- Conduct rituals or customs
- Ensure IV access patency
- Ensure medication availability

Pre-medication: Is Patient Conscious?

Yes
Does the patient report or display distress?

No
Does the patient display signs of distress?

Yes
Premedicate

No
Is patient likely to experience distress?

Yes
Premedicate?

No
Proceed to ventilator withdrawal

Yes
Premedicate

No
Proceed to ventilator withdrawal

Ventilator withdrawal algorithm.

**Ventilator Withdrawal Method:
Will Patient Initiate Spontaneous Breaths?**

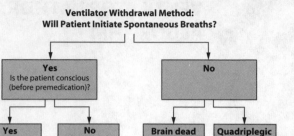

**Extubation: What Type of Airway
Does the Patient Have?**

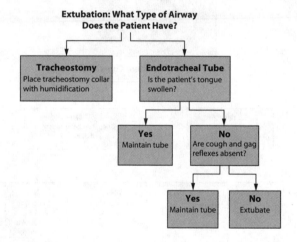

Index

Page numbers followed by *f* or *t* indicate figures or tables, respectively.